Reinventing Care

Reinventing Care

*Assisted Living
in New York City*

David Barton Smith

VANDERBILT UNIVERSITY PRESS

NASHVILLE

© 2003 Vanderbilt University Press
All rights reserved
First Edition 2003

This book is printed on acid-free paper.

Library of Congress Cataloging-in-Publication Data

Smith, David Barton.
Reinventing care : assisted living in New York City / David Barton Smith.— 1st ed.
   p. ; cm.
   Includes bibliographical references and index.
   ISBN 0-8265-1428-6 (cloth : alk. paper)
   ISBN 0-8265-1429-4 (paper : alk. paper)
   1. Aged—Long-term care—New York (State)—New York. [DNLM: 1. Assisted Living Facilities—Aged—New York City. 2. Long-Term Care—Aged—New York City. 3. Health Services for the Aged—organization & administration—New York City. WT 27 AN7 S645r 2003] I. Title.
RA564.8.S63 2003
362.1'6'097471—dc21   2003002248

*To my parents, Nancy and Henry,
to their struggle to maintain control over their lives,
and to my siblings Barbara and Woollcott
who have fought for them.*

Contents

Preface   ix

**Part I
Inventing Care**

1   Growing Old in a City   3
2   A Brief History of Care   28
3   Emergence of the Killer Application   58

**Part II
The Struggle for Control
over Markets and Lives**

4   Markets, Margin, and Mission   83
5   Private-Pay Assisted Living   98
6   Publicly Supported Assisted Living   134

**Part III
Reinventing Care**

7   A Future for Care   165

Epilogue   187

Bibliography   191

Index   199

Preface

The long-term care system frustrates the frail elderly who want to control their lives. It also frustrates those who struggle to finance, regulate, and provide their care. This book attempts to make sense of the dramatic changes in such care. It raises troubling questions about where we are headed.

The book focuses on the evolving system of care in urban America that serves more than three quarters of the nation's elderly (Eberhardt et al. 2001, 92–93). I use the New York metropolitan area to illustrate that system of care. New York City is an ideal laboratory for exploring the alternative futures of long-term care. There are an infinite variety of ways to care for the elderly in New York City. The city encompasses the largest, most concentrated population of elderly in the world. It spends more per person caring for its elderly than any other urban area. The almost one million elderly within its borders encompass the extremes of wealth and poverty. They include the residents enjoying the amenities of $10 million penthouses overlooking Central Park and those struggling just to survive in public housing units in the South Bronx. New York is the ideological capital of the world's free market. Yet many of its residents are profoundly skeptical of the ability of the market to care for the city's own elderly residents. The city has created the largest public hospital and housing system in the country and the largest concentration of voluntary philanthropic endeavors and cooperative housing arrangements in the world. Extremes provide a way of clarifying issues about how to organize care. In New York City the extremes thrive side by side. It is the major battleground where individualistic market ideology now vies with communitarian instincts to reinvent care.

Long-term care is indeed changing in the United States. The median age of nursing homes, which encompass more than 1.8 million beds, is over twenty years (Gabrel 2000, 2). Many can no longer accommodate the changing needs and expectations of residents and their families. Five of the seven largest nursing home chains operated under Chapter 11 bankruptcy protection as the new century began. Those bankruptcies affect 1,651 nursing homes and more than 200,000 residents. The market value of the stock of the ten largest nursing home companies dropped by almost $12 billion dollars, or 87%, between January 1998 and May 2000 (Dobson 2000, 20). Some might dismiss such financial news as mere bumps in the road for an industry dependent on public financing but whose long-term growth and financial viability is guaranteed by the growth of the elderly population in the United States. However, recent utilization patterns defy this assumption. The percentage of persons over sixty-five living in nursing homes in the United States dropped from 6.2% in 1982 to 3.4% in 1999 (Manton et al. 2001, 6356). Declining disability among the elderly and not just shifting patterns of use played a role in these drops (Manton et al. 1997). Something is happening. Will nursing homes be replaced, and if so, with what? Who will own what emerges and whom will they serve? How will the long-term care system that emerges shape the quality of the lives of the elderly and our society as a whole?

Future economic disparities among the elderly and our willingness to allow those disparities to dictate the care they receive will determine how the long-term care system evolves. The gaps between the rich and poor are largest in urban areas and larger still among their elderly residents (U.S. Census Bureau 1998; Rubin et al. 2000). The gulf between the rich and poor urban elderly and the care they receive is widening.

A growing body of research suggests that, rich or poor, we all have a stake in reducing those disparities. Economic inequalities adversely affect health, and relative affluence offers only limited insulation from inadequate care (Auerbach and Krimgold 2001; Mancinko and Starfield 2001). Some argue that the private security and personal services that affluence offers the elderly in urban high-rises or suburban gated communities are poor substitutes for viable community life. They support their argument with data that show that populations with lower income inequalities had longer life expectancies (Kennedy et al. 1996; Wilkinson 1996; Lynch et al. 1998). This book explores the possible implications of these conclusions for long-term care.

It is, however, not a simple story to tell. I have been influenced by the literature on the theory of complexity that is forcing a rethinking about how care should be organized (e.g., Waldrop 1992). I have adopted some of the imagery of complexity or chaos theory in this book, but the more general reader can assess the accuracy of the story and the persuasiveness of the conclusions without delving into these sometimes cumbersome abstractions. I have also been influenced more broadly by the ideas in "hermeneutic" approaches to understanding that emphasize history and the uniqueness of experiences, which are somewhat at odds with the more traditional positivistic approaches to explanation in the social sciences (e.g., Mahajan 1992; Ferrasis 1996; Schökel 1998). As a result, I have paid particular attention to the interdependence of different parts of the system and to the historical forces shaping long-term care. I spent much time digging into the past and listening to providers of care and elderly residents.

Indeed, the story I tell in this book has been evolving in my mind for more than twenty-five years. I first became fascinated with the issues surrounding long-term care in the mid-1970s when the post-Medicare-era nursing home scandals in New York State reached their pinnacle. The book I wrote about those scandals noted:

> Perhaps we have reached a new watershed. The gradual shift from local community to professional, to state and federal control of health care has been a costly one. It has created a structure that may collapse of its own weight long before the immense gap between what exists and what is obtainable in health and health care for us is closed. In the process of solving problems we have created others. Perhaps, in that process we have lost sight of where we want to go. (Smith 1981, 156)

I return now twenty-five years later to pick up that story where I left off.

I am indebted to many who made it possible to return. This book would not have been possible without the generous support of the Fan Fox and Leslie R. Samuels Foundation and a study leave from the Fox School of Business and Management at Temple University. I am especially indebted to Mary Jane Koren, then at the Fan Fox and Leslie R. Samuels Foundation and now at the Commonwealth Fund, who facilitated the organization of the three-year assisted living project, this book being one of its products. Mary Jane provided constant encouragement and guidance based on her own extensive experience in improving nursing home care as both a regulator and researcher. She was also audacious enough to serve as a marriage broker, linking me up with two remarkable individuals, Cynthia Rudder, director of the Nursing Home Community Coalition of New York State, and Geoff Lieberman, director of the Coalition of Institutionalized Aged and Disabled; the consumer advocacy groups of which they are leaders have played a key role in improving care for nursing home patients in New York State and in adult homes in New York City that care for the frail elderly and long-term psychiatric patients. I learned more through my association with these two brassy, passionate advocates than I could possibly have learned in any other way. Over the three-year course of the project, we grew to be close friends and colleagues. I am especially indebted to Cynthia and Geoff for their help in jointly conducting the case study fieldwork. Many of their observations and insights found their way into the case study chapters of this book.

This book also benefited immeasurably from the distinguished group of practitioners, researchers, and policy makers who served as the advisory group for the Fan Fox and Leslie R. Samuels Foundation Assisted Living Project. They assisted in identifying sources of information and key contacts, facilitated the design of the fieldwork, and reviewed many of the early drafts of sections of this book. The advisory group members include: William Barker, professor of preventive medicine and gerontology at the University of Rochester; Marlene Chasson, former executive director of the Friends of Residents in Long-Term Care of Raleigh, North Carolina; Holly Michaels Fisher, vice president of Visiting Nurse Service of New York; Herbert J. Horowitz, managing director of Shattuck Hammond Partners, New York; Kevin Hunter, regional president of Sunrise Assisted Living; Robert Mollica, deputy director of the National Academy for State Health Policy; Benay Phillips, chief executive officer of the Madison York Assisted Living Program; John Richter, director of Assisted Living and Community Service Policy for the New York Association of Homes and Services for the Aging; Michael Sparer, associate professor at the Columbia University School of Public Health; and Sue Reinhard of the Center for Medicare Education in Washington, D.C.

I am also indebted to the more than one hundred individuals I interviewed and checked facts with in drafting this manuscript. I am particularly indebted to the assistance of the Empire State Home and Assisted Living Association of New York State and the New York Association of Homes and Services for the Aging for encouraging their members to participate in the project. Staff of the Assisted Living Federation of America were also most helpful in guiding my inquiries. I was encouraged by the openness, graciousness, and enthusiasm of almost all of those whom I talked with. It speaks well for the emerging assisted living industry.

A special note of appreciation is also due to my colleagues and graduate students at Temple University with whom I shared and got feedback on many of the ideas that went into this book. I am especially indebted to colleagues Tom Getzen and Jackie Zinn, who reviewed and gave helpful suggestions on early drafts of the manuscript.

Old friends lightened the burden and helped improve various drafts of the manuscript. Robert Pickard provided invaluable assistance tracking down data and sources. Bruce Macleod did a careful professional editing of an early draft of the manuscript that added to the clarity of the presentation. Michael Ames, Vanderbilt University Press editor, provided a fresh pair of eyes and a perfect mix of encouragement and criticism in the final stages. Special affectionate thanks is due my wife, Joan Apt, who patiently reviewed and offered insightful suggestions throughout all the many stages of this project, as she has with other projects going back to my first book about nursing home regulation in 1981.

This book, with the kind and thoughtful help of all of these organizations and individuals, is the story of how assisted living has changed long-term care. The book is divided into three parts.

Part I sets the stage. Chapter 1 describes how care is organized for those who are growing old in New York City. The size of the city's long-term care system boggles the mind, but it consists of all the same components that exist in all metropolitan areas of the United States. The only thing that is really unique about New York's long-term care system is its own view of its uniqueness. Chapter 2 summarizes the essential historical background. It describes the invention of the current system of care and how it has been shaped by persistent tensions from the very beginnings of the city over how to best provide for and control the poor. Chapter 3 brings that history up to date and describes the emergence of assisted living, comparing it to a "killer application." A killer application in computer software is one that combines the functions of stand-alone applications but does them better and costs less. The assisted living model promises shelter, health care, control, and a real home from which, barring a medical emergency, a resident will never need to move. The promise of this model threatens the survival of some traditional health and social service organizations that provide care for a segment of a continuum of needs and those that attempt to provide care for all regardless of their ability to pay.

Part II looks inside such arrangements and describes how well facilities that claim to be providing assisted living actually deliver on their promises. This part of the book uses information gleaned from field visits to assisted living facilities done as a part of the Fan Fox and Leslie R. Samuels Foundation Assisted Living Project in collaboration with Cynthia Rudder and Geoff Lieberman. We selected ten facilities that captured much of the diversity in assisted living in New York. These included five facilities that catered exclusively to the self-pay market, both publicly traded and privately owned, and five that served those whose care was paid for almost exclusively by public sources. In this mix of facilities, we included ones with all of the different types of state licenses (enriched housing, adult homes, and assisted living programs) as well as the unlicensed "look-alikes." Since the urban market for assisted living overflows into the suburbs, we included some suburban facilities. In addition, since New York City is always accused of being a complete anachronism devoid of generalization to anywhere else and because of the extreme political, social, and economic divide between the New York metropolitan area and the rest of the state that shapes state policies that affect the city, we include some upstate facilities as well.

We provided each of these facilities with a $1,000 donation for programs and services for their residents in an effort to compensate them for the two-day disruption in their normal routines, but this would hardly have compensated them for their time. The provider associations helped identify what they considered good candidates, and few of these refused to agree to participate. As one would expect, these were all well-run facilities with no skeletons in their closets, or at least none that we could find. Nevertheless, having a pair of individuals with our backgrounds descend on them for two days armed with tape recorders and notepads, requesting lengthy interviews with key staff, access to various documents, focus groups with staff and residents, and follow-up calls to the family members of residents certainly gave them reason to hesitate before agreeing to participate. While these facilities may not be representative of facilities as a whole, we found an openness and interest in learning that speaks well for the industry as a whole. I doubt that we would have had the same success in gaining the cooperation of hospitals or nursing homes for a similar type of project.

Chapter 4 describes how, in general, such facilities work as businesses and how they attempt to achieve their somewhat contradictory mission. Unlike hospitals and nursing homes that benefit from the nearly universal coverage of the elderly offered by Medicare and Medicaid, assisted living is divided into two camps. Private-pay facilities market to, admit, and keep only those who can afford to pay their private rates. In contrast, public-pay facilities accept residents who can't pay for their care and therefore must operate on far more limited public payments.

Chapter 5 focuses on the five case study facilities that provide care exclusively to the private-pay market and explores how well each succeeds as a business and in realizing the promise of assisted living. I review how social perceptions of class and privilege influence the accomplishment of these two goals.

Chapter 6 looks at how well the five case study assisted living facilities that depend on public payments match what has been accomplished in the private market. I explore how social perceptions about community influence their success.

Part III, consisting of the final chapter, tries to distill the lessons from this analysis for policy makers, operators, and consumers. It suggests the key targets of opportunity offered by the emergence of assisted living that can improve the lives of frail seniors.

This book about assisted living is a story connected to many other important ones. Indeed, that is what makes this particular story such a fascinating one to tell.

Part I
Inventing Care

1
Growing Old in a City

> Life . . . is a sort of splendid torch which I have got a hold of for the moment, and I want to make it burn as brightly as possible before handing it on to future generations . . . the true joy in life, being used for a purpose recognized by yourself as a mighty one; the being thoroughly worn out before you are thrown on the scrap heap, being a force of nature instead of a feverish, selfish, little clod of ailments and grievances complaining that the world will not devote itself to making you happy.
> —George Bernard Shaw, *Man and Superman*

How does one grow old in a city? Many New Yorkers, and residents of other major metropolitan areas, might say that you don't. Instead, they might say that in such a place you live a full life, like that which Shaw describes in *Man and Superman*, full of the energy of a center of such lives.

For the out-of-towner, growing old or, in the language of gerontology, "aging in place," in New York City may seem absurd. The more than 30 million visitors who flood New York City each year (Better Business Bureau 2002), rubbing shoulders with its 7.4 million inhabitants, may find it an exciting place to visit, but they may also wonder why one would choose to grow old in New York City. Why, in particular, would one choose to remain in the city when just managing the simple tasks of daily living requires the caring and kindness of strangers, and quiet space for leisurely living and perhaps even the kindness of strangers are in more ample supply elsewhere? Some elderly New Yorkers do leave, but most New Yorkers live out their lives in the city. They do so not as a result of conscious decision but as a consequence of simply continuing to live their own lives.

So it is with the way care is organized for the frail elderly in New York City or anywhere else. There is no central master plan. The elderly and the informal and formal providers of their care simply invent ways to deal with the immediate circumstances they face. This chapter catalogs the pieces that make up the large, constantly evolving, complex system that cares for the frail elderly in New York City: the population that system serves, the providers caring for that population, and the ways their care is paid for.

The Population

Migration and dependency patterns determine how many people need long-term care in New York City. There are about one million people over the age of sixty-five living in the city's five boroughs (Claritas 1998). About one third of them live alone, and more than one fifth have mobility and self-care needs. The more than 139,000 persons in New York City over the age of eighty-five comprise the largest portion of those with mobility and self-care needs and of those who reside in nursing homes. In the United States as a whole, those over eighty-five are the most rapidly growing age group. In New York City, the eighty-five-plus population grew by 10% over the last five years.

The financial resources of New York City's elderly determine the kind of care they are able to receive. About 63% of households over sixty-five in 1990 in New York City had household incomes of less than $25,000 per year, far less than the annual cost of personal care.

The ethnic diversity of the city shapes the availability of informal family caregivers and the character of the formal care that is provided. Foreign-born and second-generation immigrants account for 60% of New York City's population. Blacks, Hispanics, Asians, and nonnative persons accounted for 84% of the city's population in 1998 (Waters et al. 1999). Immigrants provide more than half of the formal direct care for frail elderly residents in New York City. It is easier for them to find work in direct care than in other fields. The nature of the work is more familiar to many immigrants than other kinds of employment, and the low wages make such jobs easier to get than higher-paying jobs. Home health aides and personal care assistants from Nigeria, Haiti, Ghana, and India tend to cluster together in individual facilities.

One cannot begin to understand the system of long-term care in New York or that of the nation as whole without understanding the effect of elderly migration patterns. The elderly migrating from New York City include high-income individuals with plenty of options and middle-income individuals who are no longer able to afford the rising cost of living in the city. They become part of the "hollowing out" of its upper- and middle-income population. Many urban policy makers fear that a combination of rising tax burdens and declining services might accelerate this trend into a death spiral as it has in other urban areas (McMahon et al. 1997). Younger, poorer families have limited possibilities for home ownership, but older, middle-income residents are homeowners and can sell their property and use the capital to find attractive alternatives at a lower cost in the Sunbelt. Some keep their New York City residences as investments, anticipating higher prices in the future, and they join the seasonal "snowbirds" who travel south in the winter (Hogan and Steimes 1992).

In general, migration follows the stages of the life cycle. Migration rates rise as adults enter stable employment between the ages of twenty and forty. It then declines. There is a small jump in migration rates at retirement ages, and then it slopes upward again with increasing age. Real estate agents have the greatest opportunity to sell a residence to an individual or family during three transition periods of people's lives: when they gain new employment, when they reach retirement, and as they face the growing frailties of old age. The "retirement peak" and the upward "late age slope" represent two distinct parts of the so-called senior housing market. Economic considerations, duration of residence, location of family members, climate, and availability of health services influence seniors' relocation decisions (Kallan 1993).

The net migration of the elderly out of New York City leaves it with a sicker and poorer population to care for. New York State ranks second among the states in net elderly migration rate. (Alaska with its even more inhospitable winters and high cost of living ranks first.) The ratio of elderly out-migration to in-migration is more than 8 to 1. New York City's five counties all rank within the top fifteen counties in the nation in ratio of out-migration to in-migration, with Queens and Kings being second and third, outranked only by Nassau County, New York. Similar patterns exist in most large northern cities in the United States. Net migration out of New York State resulted in a 6.4% reduction in the over-sixty population in the city between 1985 and 1990 (calculated from 1990 U.S. Census and Longino 1995). Net migration out of the city to other parts of the state is roughly equivalent. In New York State as a whole, out-migration was offset during this period by a 27.4% growth in the elderly population through aging of existing residents. In addition, immigration of elderly from abroad produced a 1% increase (Frey 1995, 764). In 1990 the New York State population over sixty stood at 3.2 million, the largest elderly population of any state, followed closely only by Florida, with a 1990 elderly population of 3.0 million. New York and Florida also have the largest exchange of citizens over the age of sixty. Florida was the destination of 21% of the New York State's elderly migrants, and New York was the destination of 47% of Florida's. Many of the elderly who migrate from Florida to New York are New Yorkers who had moved to Florida earlier in their retirement and return to New York in the final years of their lives. It was a common story I heard from residents, family members, and staff at elderly care facilities in New York.

The economic impact of these elderly migration patterns on both Florida and New York is staggering. For New Yorkers, the most popular destinations are the South Florida counties of Broward, Palm Beach, and Dade. New York ranks dead last among the states in economic impact from elderly migration, with a net loss of $3.3 billion per year in elderly household income; Florida ranks first, with a net gain as a result of in-migration of $6.5 billion per year (Longino 1995, 85). Migration directly from New York accounts for more than $1.8 billion of Florida's net gain. Given the generally higher income levels of New York City residents and the fact that they account for almost half of all migration out of the state, more than half of the state's losses accrue directly to the city. These figures do not account for the transfer of wealth, volunteer services, and support of religious and cultural activities that the added leisure of retirement brings (Kim and Hong 1998). They also do not take into account the adverse effect on New York of the loss of healthy and more affluent older citizens due to migration. In effect, this leaves an elderly population in New York City more in need of medical services but less able to afford the out-of-pocket costs. For example, corrected for age differences, the per capita Medicare costs alone for New York City's five boroughs are among the highest of any counties in the nation. Some of these cost differences are shaped by the migration and return migration patterns. In health insurance terminology, New York is a victim of regional "adverse risk selection."

Like the insurance practice that state insurance commissioners attempt to prevent, Sunbelt states such as Florida, and particularly the South Florida counties of Dade, Broward, and Palm Beach, engage in unabashed, predatory regional "cream skimming." Their explicit development strategy is to keep the tax rates low to encourage immigration by offering more affordable retirement conditions while at the same time limiting services to encourage reverse migration when an elderly individual has exhausted his or her own resources and requires subsidized services such as Medicaid nursing home care (Berry and Henrietta 1996). Florida, unlike New York, has no state income, estate, or death taxes. Medical services, prescriptions, and groceries are exempt from Florida's 7% sales tax. Florida's Medicaid program spends less per elderly resident than New York—$340 in contrast to New York's $2,640—and less per elderly Medicaid enrollee, $4,479 in contrast to New York's $17,101 (Holahan et al. 1998, 39). New York has the highest per capita Medicaid expenditure of any state for long-term care, and Florida has one of the lowest. In addition, Florida's long-term care expenditures are devoted exclusively to nursing facilities (94.5%), while 25.3% of New York's long-term care expenditures go for home care. (This difference will take on more significance in the light of the history of such care described in the next chapter.) Florida's elderly are healthier and less impaired than those in other states, and they have greater financial resources (Berry and Henrietta 1996).

Broward County draws the largest number of elderly migrants from New York City to Florida. Its sprawling metropolitan area of Fort Lauderdale now encompasses a population of more than 1.58 million. More than 256,000 are over the age of sixty-five, the majority having moved to Broward after retirement. The retirement developments that they inhabit are a major engine driving the rapid growth and economic development of the county. Fort Lauderdale has no real downtown or center as do northeastern cities such as New York, where major growth came before the automobile-spawned suburban sprawl after World War II. The developments spread like high-tide marks on a beach. Most of the older developments of the 1960s and 70s abut each other in townships close to the shore. Many of the inhabitants, like the buildings in these communities, have aged in place and are in decline. The newer developments that attract more recent retirees are further inland, pushing up against the Everglades. Open land for new developments has shrunk, as have the orange groves and winter vegetable farms that used to be the dominant force in the local economy before the 1960s. As land prices have risen, developers have bulldozed the older, more affordable trailer park communities to make way for higher-priced condominiums. This has forced a new wave of migration of the longtime year-round residents and snowbirds who had put down roots in those developments.

For more affluent elderly New Yorkers, Broward County offers luxury gated communities with twenty-four-hour security and roving patrols. The price tags range from $300,000 to well over $1 million. In neighboring Palm Beach and Dade Counties the prices for residences in such new luxury developments can rise to as high as $10 million. The amenities include golf courses, tennis courts, boat-docking slips, and orange groves.

Broward County still offers relatively affordable housing for the majority of New York's expatriate retirees who seek homes to match their more modest retirement budgets. Attractive manufactured homes in "active adult communities" with several baths and bedrooms, pleasant grounds with orange groves, and a clubhouse run between $30,000 and $80,000.

Mobile home parks, at the low end of the retirement housing market, once represented a major and even dominant form of housing in some of Broward County's municipalities. The prices of these homes range from $15,000 to as much as $50,000. The parks can be set up by a developer with the purchase or lease of vacant land and a modest investment in providing water, sewage, and a septic system. One can then attach a bucolic name to a few acres with palm trees and scrub brush and be open for business. As one northern émigré observer noted,

> If a sales organization digs a hole in the ground in order to get fill for home building, suddenly there is a lake that can lend a name to the development. Westwind Lakes or Pinecrest Lakes are two that come to mind. Where I was raised, the folks sometimes named a body of water after its color. I remember one spot called "Mud Lake." That would never happen in Florida. Ocean Pavilion, King's Creek and River Shores are typical names given to water front dwellings awaiting elderly fugitives from urban squalor. . . . The homes are villas as in Shadywood Villas, never Cracker Box houses. This is understandable. We worked all our lives and want to live in places called King Court or Coral Reef Estates. Royal Glen has a nice ring to it. Why settle for Jensen Bog? (Jensen 1987)

Many of the mobile homes were settled by snowbirds who followed the winter migration south and slowly took up roots in their Broward County winter residencies. Rising land prices, growing affluence, and the shrinkage of undeveloped land in the county now threaten the mobile home parks with extinction. The older ones began closing in the 1980s. Operators were unwilling to make the investments necessary to meet stricter housing code standards on the homes and to maintain facilities on which time and weather had taken their toll. For many residents of these older mobile homes, moving the trailer was not an option. The trailer owners in some parks battled back. Many had honed their skills earlier in their lives battling landlords in New York City. They organized and won temporary legal and political victories but eventually succumbed to more powerful economic forces and their own growing frailty. One of the remaining struggles now involves a mobile home park leased on Seminole land that the tribe now plans to use to build a gambling casino complex, including a Hard Rock Café (Vise and Bolstad 2000).

No matter what the income bracket, the housing developments and their local municipalities struggle to deal with the aging in place of their residents. Managers of the housing complexes may see the growing frailty and disorientation of a resident and notify the municipal governments, many of whom have hired outreach workers, often retirees themselves, to visit and check up on residents. In many cases, this will trigger a search for adult children and other relatives. Phone calls will bring family members down from New York, and this will often result in reverse migration. Many struggle not just with their growing frailty but also with the death of a spouse and with the unanticipated rising costs of living in South Florida. Those events may also trigger a return to New York City to be close to their adult children.

Broward County as a whole struggles to meet the growing needs of the most rapidly growing segment of the population, the more than 35,000 residents over the age of eighty-five. The Area Agency on Aging reports long waiting lists of more than 1,400 individuals for in-home personal care services. Thus Broward County, like other Sunbelt destinations, skims the cream. Such communities draw the well and more affluent elderly as an engine for their own regional growth, attracting them with their lower taxes and sometimes necessitating their return when subsidies for home care and nursing care that higher tax rates should provide prove absent. It is, however, an engine for economic growth that some Floridians view with ambivalence. Getting the tax increases necessary to improve long-term care and supportive services for the frail elderly is not a high priority on the state's political agenda.

While this migration pattern has a significant impact on New York City, the overwhelming majority of the city's elderly, like the elderly everywhere else, never make such treks in the first place. More than 85% never leave the city. Most would regard the possibility of relocation to

Florida with disdain. "The best place to retire," observed the head of the International Longevity Center, Robert N. Butler (a New York City resident in his late seventies, but hardly retired), "is the neighborhood where you spent your life" (Boyer 1987). They remain a part of the fabric of local neighborhoods, accounting for more than their share of attendance at the city's sporting events, neighborhood restaurants, churches and synagogues, and cultural events. Just as elsewhere, most frail elderly stay where they are, tied by habit, the comforts of navigating familiar physical surroundings, family, and friendships. They harbor the stubborn resistance to the stigma implied by retirement relocation and, as a consequence, depend on the care available in the city.

The Providers

In his 1999 state of the city address, City Council Speaker Peter Vallone spoke to the need for providing the services that the city's elderly require:

> Some people mistakenly believe New York is a place where people live until they move to Miami. I don't accept that idea. When I hear someone is moving south, I want it to be South Brooklyn, the South Bronx and South Ozone Park. Now, I don't want to start a war with Florida. It's a great place to visit.... I just wouldn't want to live there. Nothing beats the stimulation and excitement of living in a great city. To be in New York City is to be involved in life ... to be part of today, not yesterday. Regrettably, many seniors who would like to stay in New York find themselves forced out by a shortage of affordable senior housing. And that's a shame. Literally. Shame on all of us.... Many apartment complexes in our City now have a significant number of older residents. These are known as Naturally Occurring Retirement Communities or NORCs. In New York City over 350,000 seniors live in such neighborhoods. They want to stay in the City, but often find it difficult to live independently. We have to look beyond senior centers and provide these older people with the services they urgently need.
> ... What do we owe to our seniors? That's easy. We owe them everything. We owe them care. We owe them love. We owe them life. And one more thing. We owe them the survival of our nation. (Vallone 1999)

Most of those whom Vallone referred to, those who weathered the Great Depression in childhood and helped bring World War II to a successful conclusion, stay and age in place in New York City. As they age, they begin to navigate a complex network of services in the city. That network includes four distinct layers of increasingly institutionalized and medicalized care: (1) independent living or self-organized care, (2) sheltered housing, (3) nursing homes, and (4) acute care hospitals.

Independent Living and Self-Organized Care

While New York City seems a hostile environment for the frail elderly, as do most large urban areas, it hides a rich complexity of arrangements that make independent living for many of its frail elderly residents almost idyllic. As City Council Speaker Vallone noted, more than 350,000 New Yorkers over the age of sixty live in naturally occurring retirement communities (NORCs). The term, coined in 1985, generally identifies apartment complexes and residential blocks where over 50% of the residents are fifty or older (Hunt and Gunter-Hunt 1985). They are not apartment complexes or neighborhoods designed for this purpose. They just happen. There are two ways they happen. They can happen through relocation, as in the case of many municipalities in Broward County, or they can happen through "aging in place," as in the case of New York City. Patterns similar to those in New York City develop anywhere new housing complexes open up and leave clusters of older residents in the older complexes in the area. Almost half of the low- and moderate-income apartment buildings constructed with government assistance in New York City have become NORCs. There are 141 publicly supported moderate- and middle-income rental and limited-equity cooperative developments in New York City, with approximately 52,761 apartment units. (The "limited equity" cooperatives restrict the amount owners can receive from the sale of their apartment.) In addition, there are another 240,245 cooperative or condominium apartments in non–publicly sponsored apartment complexes in the city. Rent control applies to all buildings in New York City constructed before 1947 and to those who have been living in their apartments continuously since 1971. Tenants over the age of sixty-two who live in rent-controlled or -stabilized apartments are entitled to exemption from rental increases if they are below certain income thresholds. Not surprisingly, persons over the age of sixty-five occupy 41,000 rent-controlled apartments in New York City, or about 59% of all such apartments in the city. The median age of householders in the publicly supported housing cooperatives is fifty-four, and 28.7% are over age sixty-five. The cooperative ownership arrangements and the city's rent-control laws offer powerful incentives for aging in place and for the development of NORCs.

Informal caregivers play an essential role in making NORCs work. They make it possible for the frail elderly to continue to live outside of the formal care system. A survey of such providers in New York City indicates that they are most typically the daughter of the frail elderly person; that they provide, on average, twenty hours of care a week; and that almost half have been providing such care for more than five years (Levine 2000). Most do so on their own without additional paid help. They provide assistance with activities of daily living (bathing, dressing, feeding, incontinence, ambulation) and with medications. This invisible part of the health care economy in New York City, as elsewhere, far outnumbers the more visible formal health care sector. A "midrange estimate" places the number of such informal caregivers at 25.8 million nationally and the total value of their services at $196 billion, almost twice the national expenditure for nursing home and professional home care services (Arno and Levine 1999).

For well-heeled New Yorkers, the services in such NORCs are unparalleled. An apartment dweller on the Upper East Side can have dinner from an almost unlimited exotic array of restaurant take-outs delivered to their door in less than half an hour. A solicitous doorman looks out for their welfare, assures security, and arranges transportation and the delivery of any services desired. The expertise of the world's largest concentration of medical specialists and researchers and the stimulation of the world's largest concentration of cultural attractions are a five-minute cab ride away. Indeed, a *Business Week* feature even promoted New York City as one of the "urban hot spots" for those seeking a retirement relocation where "being near the fifth hole isn't enough" (Baig and Reiss 1998).

For those who revel in the intellectual energy of the city but have limited resources, local groups have created inventive solutions. Morningside Gardens on West 123rd Street, for example, houses two thousand residents in six twenty-story towers on ten acres. Columbia University, Barnard College, Bank Street College of Education, the Jewish Theological Seminary, and the Union Theological Seminary along with local churches formed a corporation and with federal and state financial assistance built Morningside, which opened in 1957. By the mid-1980s more than half the residents were over the age of sixty-five. Morningside began experiencing all the predictable but never-planned-for problems of NORCs.

There was the recluse whose apartment began to exude foul odors, the wandering elderly resident with dementia, and the aging alcoholic whose wife locked him out when he got drunk. In 1986 the co-op governing body created Morningside Retirement and Health Services and, with some seed money from a foundation, hired a social worker to help facilitate services for residents. Those services have now expanded to include two full-time social workers, a music therapy group, a home health aid, shopping and escort services, visits by geriatric residents from a local hospital, cultural field trips, a Medicare clinic for expediting residents' insurance paperwork, blood pressure testing and monitoring, a weekly movie program, and a writing workshop. The writing workshop, conducted by Columbia faculty member and novelist Mary Gordon, typically has about fifteen active members. Eileen Tobin, one of the workshop's early participants published short stories in a literary magazine for the first time in 1997 and, in 2000, at the age of eighty-five, she had one of her stories published in an anthology of older women writers entitled *Crimson Edge: Older Women Writing*. The phrase "Crimson Edge" in the title, as its editor Sondra Zeidenstein explains, represents the thin red line on the horizon at sunset. "But it does more than signal that the day is fading," she says; it "reconfigures the sky" (Haberman 2000).

For average retired working people—teachers, social workers, and blue-collar workers with union pension plans—some of the other co-op apartment complexes in the city cannot be matched. The Penn South Mutual Redevelopment Houses lie just south of Penn Station on the west side of Manhattan. This moderate-income cooperative complex opened in 1962. Many of the current six thousand residents moved in when it opened. Over 75% of the residents are now over sixty-five. "Living here is a very special thing. It's like living in a small town where everybody knows each other just a few blocks from Broadway and Greenwich Village," observed one of the more active co-op members. Like Morningside's, the Penn South co-op's board members saw a growing need for services to care for their aging members. They surveyed the wishes of the residents, sought funding, and recruited service partners. A program evolved that included group activities, volunteer programs, case management, and home care coordination. The size and concentration of this elderly population as well as the organizing skills of its leadership (it included retired social workers and organizers for the International Ladies' Garment Workers' Union) attracted partners. They have partnered with the Visiting Nurse Service of New York, which saw the opportunity to find Medicare- and Medicaid-reimbursable cases while providing free care to residents through a satellite office in the senior center. Beth Israel Hospital opened geriatric medical practices and offers "free" flu shots, lectures, and screenings for the residents. Saint Vincent's, a psychiatric facility, has also partnered with the co-op and provides cognitive assessments and more specialized mental health services to residents. In addition, the Penn South program for seniors has been successful in getting both city and state appropriations for its activities and those of similar NORCs. The retired organizers of the co-op program have now launched new careers as consultants to other co-op housing projects both in New York and nationally and are busy developing an assisted living expansion to serve the residents of Penn South.

The more fortunate low-income elderly have aged in place in the public housing projects located in the safer neighborhoods with more fashionable addresses. They have a strong informal network of neighborhood friends and a growing array of supportive services. The New York City Housing Authority's 346 developments and 181,000 apartment units are home to approximately 535,000 residents (New York City Housing Authority 2001). The size of the operation is hard to comprehend. If it were a city, it would rank as the twenty-second largest in the United States. It is three times the size of Chicago's housing authority, the second largest. The New York City Housing Authority receives about 70% of its $2.4 billion in annual revenues from the federal government, 28% from tenant rents, and the remaining 2% from New York State. Historically, like public housing programs in many other parts of the country, it has provided homes predominantly for the working poor. These developments began to be built in the 1930s and were built to last. None have been torn down, and they are generally well maintained. "We have served as the anchor and cornerstone in some of the lower-income neighborhoods and some, such as some of the developments on the Lower East Side, have helped revitalize the area," said one administrator I interviewed. Most who move in never leave. No new developments have been constructed since 1980. The average length of residence is seventeen years, and 34% or 61,000 of the heads of households in the developments are over the age of sixty. Only 7,100 seniors live in specifically designated senior housing developments, with the bulk aging in place in the family units of the housing authority's developments. "There's an incredible informal network among the seniors; they look after each other and go into each other's apartments to make sure everything is okay. The apartment managers are a part of that network of services," the same administrator said.

Just as they have in higher-income apartment complexes with a growing concentration of elderly, services have sprung up in response to the needs of elderly housing authority tenants. A senior resident advisor program began as a demonstration in the housing authority in 1979 and has since become nationally recognized. It provides a free apartment and modest salary to individuals who agree to be on call twenty-four hours a day to assist elderly residents with problems and coordinate services for them. The program currently provides on-site services for 5,200 seniors in twenty-two developments. In addition, the housing authority operates forty senior centers that organize preventive health programs and activities for seniors in its developments. Seven of the twenty-eight NORCs in the city that are now officially recognized with state and city funds to support the organization of services operate in the housing authority's developments. The funds support outreach and social workers. Like the other NORCs, most have begun to develop partnerships with health care providers for on-site services that can be covered by Medicaid and Medicare.

The home health services that Medicaid covers in New York State make it possible to envision the low-income NORCs evolving into full-blown assisted living facilities. The coverage of home health services by Medicaid is the most distinctive feature of the health care system in New York, which in other respects is quite similar to that of other states. New York State provides the most extensive and costly Medicaid package of home care benefits of any state. It provides both short-term home health care for patients discharged from a hospital and home attendant care for the chronically ill. Currently about half of what is spent nationally in the Medicaid program for such care is spent in New York State. In 1998 this amounted to almost $2.4 billion, with 81%, or more than $1.9 billion, spent in New York City (New York State Department of Health 2000).

The Medicaid home health care program in the city serves a frail and vulnerable population. A recent survey estimates that 81% of the 65,000 Medicaid home health care recipients live in the city's fifteen poorest neighborhoods, 40% live alone, 90% suffer from at least one chronic health condition, and 75% are impaired in performing at least three basic activities of daily living, such as bathing and eating (Hokenstad et al. 1998). "Many live in isolation and fear, imprisoned in their apartments.

Maybe half would benefit with assistance in getting groceries or preparing meals. Depression, alcohol abuse, and suicide are common problems," one home health agency administrator said. Those whose assets or income disqualifies them for Medicaid but who cannot afford to pay out of pocket for services represent a major impediment faced by the housing authority in developing functional full-service NORCs. As one elderly resident observed, "I've worked every day of my life, and Mrs. Fisher never worked one. She's got a personal care aide that comes in to help her. Why can't I have one?" Many could ask similar questions, particularly those who feel forced to choose between filling prescriptions and shopping for groceries.

However, the shortage of adequate affordable housing for the low-income population casts the largest shadow over all these supportive efforts. While many other urban areas in the United States face similar problems with access to affordable housing, New York City has faced the most extreme and persistent shortage. Housing conditions in New York City have constituted an emergency under New York State law since 1950. More than 284,000 applications flood the housing authority waiting list for public and Section 8 housing. The waiting time for housing authority apartments for those who do not become special priorities (e.g., working poor families and the homeless) now averages seventeen years. The Housing Authority also provides 77,000 families with vouchers to assist with the rental of private apartments. This is helpful if the eligible applicant already lives in an apartment that meets the standards to qualify. However, it is difficult, if not impossible, to find such low-rent apartments in the current market. Federal regulations define spending more than 30% of one's household income for housing as excessive. The median single elderly household in the New York City, before subsidies, spends 50.7% of its income on housing. Thus, most of the low-income elderly live at the bottom of the housing stock in the city, in buildings with growing maintenance and structural problems, in neighborhoods that are no longer safe. Some must painfully climb six floors to a walkup apartment that has seen brighter days. For some, a stroke, a fall, or a broken hip ends the struggle to maintain independence and the fragile network of support they had organized.

Many of the city's poor go without the care that they need. More than 13,500 received government-subsidized home-delivered meals, but the waiting lists for meals are long. For some, this single meal is supplemented with little else. Malnutrition is rampant. Some supplement their diets by foraging in garbage bins, and in a few extreme cases, some starve to death. The visits of a senior center outreach team uncover bleak conditions among those who are no longer able to live independently. They find the man with Alzheimer's disease left alone when his wife was hospitalized. They find a confused woman in a squalid apartment who has not eaten for four days. Sometimes they find the dead (Goodnough 1994). For others, larger, more powerful forces transforming the urban landscape obliterate their independence. As one 1998 focus group participant explained, "I fell down and broke my leg. While I was in the hospital, the landlord burned down the apartment building. He died of a heart attack, though, so he didn't even have the chance to collect. I had no place to go."

An epidemic of fires cresting in the middle 1970s spread through the traditional slum neighborhoods of Harlem, East Harlem, the Lower East Side, Brownsville, Bedford Stuyvesant, Williamsburg, and the South Bronx. Waves of migration and dislocations disrupted stable surrounding neighborhoods. The social dislocations spread the accompanying urban plagues of violent crime, TB, low birth-weight babies, and AIDS. The city has yet to recover from the cascading sequence of events. Public urban development policies of benign neglect and the resulting reallocation of fire department resources appear to have triggered this sequence of events (Wallace and Wallace 1998). The low-income frail elderly continue to be the major victims of these policies, slipping through the informal network of self- and family-organized supports and into the city's more formalized arrangements for care. Some end up in one of the city's remaining seventy-two single-room occupancy (SRO) hotels.

The city's press has chronicled the battle between the fixed-income elderly tenants of SRO hotels and landlords who for more than thirty years have been seeking to improve their profits by converting these hotels to tourist hotels or higher-priced condominiums. It is a story similar to the disappearance of the mobile trailer parks in Broward County but often a more brutal one. Many of the current SRO hotels were once reputable hotels and apartment complexes converted to accommodate the flood of single workers into the city during and after World War II. As the demand for apartments increased in the 1970s, many were converted to apartments and co-ops. The options for the existing tenants, often disabled or elderly with limited incomes, were few. The city imposed a moratorium on such conversions in 1983. The courts overturned it in 1989. The landlords could increase their income more than tenfold over the rent-controlled SRO rates by converting to tourist hotels or condominiums. It was a matter of making conditions sufficiently unbearable so that people who had very little other choice would leave. These existing SRO tenants cannot legally be kicked out, but as they leave or die conversions can take place. Prior to twenty years ago tenants had fewer protections. "They weren't at all subtle back then," observed one housing advocate. "They just hired goons and kicked you out" (Siegal 1999). For some, the process became only a shade subtler. The SRO hotels now range from poor but reasonably safe and clean to squalid, degrading, and dangerous. On the low end, maintenance is deferred and buildings are allowed to deteriorate. They become homes for drug addicts, prostitutes, and the mentally ill. Some SRO landlords allegedly still hire thugs to rob and terrorize tenants (Lobbia 1997).

Sheltered Housing

Together, New York City and New York State provide a bewildering variety of arrangements for more formalized sheltered housing and refuge for the more vulnerable elderly. In other states such facilities are licensed as boarding, personal care, or assisted living facilities, but the residents and the type of services they provided are much the same. Some states also provide care to nursing home–eligible residents in these facilities and by home health agencies under a Medicaid waiver program. In New York State there are three kinds of licensed facilities that provide such care: adult homes, enriched housing, and assisted living programs operated within either an adult home or an enriched housing setting. The licensed adult homes provide housing, meals, and some limited social activities and personal care to residents. There are fifty-one adult homes licensed in the city; forty are for-profit operations, and the remainder nonprofit. About half have more than 25% discharged psychiatric hospital patients mixed in with the frail elderly. In addition, there are nine enriched housing programs located in subsidized nonprofit low-income complexes that provide for a somewhat similar array of services for their elderly apartment dwellers. Ten of these licensed facilities in the city have assisted living programs (ALPs) approved for payment by the state Medicaid program that are designed to provide care for nursing home–eligible residents in conjunction with a licensed home health agency, with at total capacity of 1,056. The ALP units are entitled to Medicaid payments equivalent to half the nursing Medicaid rate for particular types of patients, in addition to Supplemental Security Income (SSI) payments. For a typical resident in an ALP unit, a "Physical A" (a patient needing relatively routine and inexpensive physical care), the facility receives a Medicaid payment of $59.65 per day. Altogether these licensed facilities in New York City have a capacity for 9,327 residents. The average size is 141 beds. They range in size from a 427-bed proprietary adult home located on Staten Island to an eleven-resident enriched housing arrangement operated by a nonprofit agency in Manhattan. In general, the facilities in the city are larger than ones located upstate and in other parts of the country. They rely almost exclusively either on private payments by residents or SSI payments. Few facilities serve both the private and SSI populations. The current SSI rate in New York for adult care facilities is $27 a day.

The licensed adult homes that rely on public payments cover the full range of conditions. Some manage through the energy and dedication of their staff and residents to create clean, warm, lively communities in Spartan surroundings. These are places in which no adult child would feel bad about leaving his or her parent. There are others, particularly those whose residents are mostly psychiatric patients, that rival the worst snake pits of the early twentieth century. One of the worst is a for-profit home housing 360 mentally ill residents that remains open despite a decade of horror stories (Levy and Kershaw 2001). In 1989 two residents of the home died under mysterious circumstances, one padlocked in a closet. In 1993 a decomposed body was found wedged behind a basement freezer. In 2000 the Health Department ordered the evacuation of residents on the first floor after an inspection found soiled linen, vermin infestation, and badly damaged walls and ceilings. In 2001 the Health Department conducted an inquiry into the assembly-line prostatectomies on twenty-four residents involving questionable appropriateness and consent. The urologist performed the surgery at one of the city's only remaining small for-profit hospitals, in which he had an ownership interest. In April 2002 the *New York Times* published a three-part series outlining similar abuses and the failure to regulate the city's adult homes adequately (Clifford 2002).

In addition, offering living arrangements to higher-income clientele, there is a largely invisible unlicensed segment. Those operating in this segment describe their facilities as assisted living or senior residential housing. They operate as a part of the private apartment market in the New York City and target the higher-income frail elderly. Monthly fees that include rent, meals, and some services in these unlicensed private facilities range between $2,000 and $6,000. Eighteen of these unlicensed facilities responded to a telephone survey developed by this study in the fall of 1999. They had a total capacity of 2,020 units. The average number of apartment units in these unlicensed facilities is 112. They have provided such care for an average of about ten years and operate at 88% of capacity overall. Thirteen of the eighteen responding facilities were nonprofits, and the remainder were for-profit operations. Most observers in 1999 forecasted explosive growth of this segment of the market from the many planned conversions of hotels and apartment buildings and new construction in progress. Some have the look and feel of luxury hotels. Atria West Side, a recently converted residential hotel on the Upper West Side of Manhattan, for example, offers a penthouse lounge and terrace gardens with spectacular views of the Manhattan skyline. Amenities include a surround-sound theater and parlors with fireplaces. Residents can, for a price, rent spacious, high-ceiling apartments with two bedrooms, two baths, a full kitchen, and private terraces with a skyline view. However, in accommodation to the city's rent-control laws, about a third of the facility's inhabitants are tenants who predate the acquisition and conversion by Atria. The tenants include couples with children and middle-aged professionals. Thus, Atria West Side offers, through no intention of its own, perhaps one of the only age-integrated assisted living facilities in the country.

At the other extreme, services now coordinated under New York City's Department of Homeless Services provide shelter for the poorest and most desperate of the city's elderly inhabitants (New York City Government 2001). Its Division of Adult Services manages 44 shelters with a capacity for over 7,500 persons. The department directly operates eight of these shelters, and the remainder are operated under contract by nonprofit social service organizations. The shelters provide temporary accommodations. Seventy-nine percent of those in these shelters are male. The average age is forty-three. Alcohol, drug addiction, and mental health problems figure prominently in this population, but many operators believe the older persons in the mental health population need most of the same assistance as the frail elderly cared for in other settings. For those living on the streets, the department operates nine drop-in centers, eight of which are under contract with nonprofit social service providers that offer social services, meals, and showers. Seven outreach teams, six under contract with nonprofit social service organizations, attempt to provide services to those living on the streets and in other public places. The objective of all these efforts is to transition this population to more permanent housing arrangements. In addition to the licensed adult homes and enriched housing mentioned above, some of the elderly in this population end up in the dwindling number of SRO hotels. Landlords renting to a homeless individual can also receive a one-time rent bonus and Section 8 subsidies up to what is defined as the fair market rate.

Those who slip through all of these sheltered housing arrangements end up filling the emergency rooms of the city's hospitals. Many have impaired and declining mental and physical conditions for which little can be done. Those who have had successful professional lives blend in with those who have lived marginal ones, sharing the universal human experiences of aging, illness, suffering, and death. They are all assigned the label GOMER (Get Out of My Emergency Room) or other pejorative terms by the frustrated young interns and residents who attend them (Leiderman and Grisso 1985). They wait together either to be admitted to the hospital, pending nursing home placement, or to be transferred directly from the emergency department to a nursing home.

Nursing Homes

There are 185 licensed nursing homes in New York's five boroughs, with a total of 43,897 beds for those who, largely for medical reasons, can't be cared for in less restrictive settings. These facilities provide twenty-four-hour skilled nursing supervision and care. They range in size from the 816-bed Jewish Home and Hospital in the Bronx and the 775-bed Coler Memorial public facility on Roosevelt Island to a 35-bed proprietary facility on Staten Island. The average size is 237 beds. Ownership of the city's nursing homes is split between proprietary (51%) and voluntary operations (44%). Seven facilities operated by the city make up the remainder. The 4.37 beds per 100 population over sixty-five in the state contrasts with 5.27 beds per 100 in the United States as a whole, and with 2.91 bed per 100 in the State of Florida. In 1997 the average occupancy rate was 98%, higher than for any other state. There were 50,433 Medicaid-eligible elderly New Yorkers who received care in those nursing homes in fiscal year 1997–98 at an average cost of $40,239 and a total cost of $2.031 billion (New York State Department of Health 2000). Unlike in most other states, Medicaid payments in New York to nursing homes compare reasonably to private rates. Concentrations of Medicaid and private residents in different facilities are more reflective of the composition of the service areas than of selective admitting practices by the facilities.

Acute Care Hospitals

There are 74 licensed acute hospitals in New York's five boroughs, with a total of 31,428 beds and an overall occupancy in the second quarter of 1998 of 69.5%. This means there are 4.26 acute hospital beds per 1,000 people in the city. Altogether both the bed population ratio and the occupancy rate in the city are slightly higher than the overall national figures (4.00 hospital beds per 1,000 and an occupancy rate in 1998 of 65%). New York's elderly were discharged from acute hospitals 298,712 times during 1998, with an average length of stay of 9.37 days. This translates into 297 discharges per 1,000 elderly persons and a total number of days per 1,000 elderly of 2,784. The hospital discharge rate for New York City's elderly residents is 20% below the national rates (297 vs. 365 per 1,000), but their average length of stay is 51% higher than the national average (9.37 vs. 6.20) (Hall and Popovic 2000, 6; New York State Department of Health 2001b). As a result New York City's elderly had a 30% higher rate of hospital days per 1,000 than the national average (2,784 vs. 2,149). In other words, the city's elderly are less likely to be admitted to a hospital but are more likely to stay longer and fill more acute hospital beds. About half return to their homes, with another 14% receiving home health care in their homes.

New York City's seventy-four acute hospitals are overwhelmingly owned by nonprofit voluntary organizations. The only significant exceptions are the eleven public hospitals operated by the city's Health and Hospitals Corporation. These public hospitals continue to have a unique and vital role in the city's health system (Opdyck 1999). This contrasts to the southern and western regions of the United States, where for-profit hospitals have a large, if not dominant, presence. The dominance of nonprofit ownership in New York reflects the history of hospital development in the Northeast and Midwest and the city's own distinctive aversion to for-profit health care. Only five small proprietary facilities are currently licensed as hospitals in the city. Major teaching hospitals and medical centers have expanded by acquiring hospitals, which created considerable consolidation of ownership in the last decade (Cantor et al. 1998). The city's hospitals struggle with growing financial problems. Sixty-one percent reported operating losses in 2000, eleven of thirty-six studied by the United Hospital Fund were in jeopardy of closing, and another nine faced serious financial problems that placed them at risk of such a fate (United Hospital Fund 2001).

Paying for Care

Paying for the care of the frail elderly in New York City is expensive, but elderly New Yorkers as a whole have a lot of resources. Table 1.1 summarizes those resources. The average income of the over-sixty-five resident is more than $25,000, and their average net worth is approximately $311,000. These resources pay for living expenses and for medical care and personal assistance not covered by health insurance. If these combined costs exceed an elderly individual or couple's income, they can liquidate their assets by selling their home or dipping into savings. The federal Medicare program pays an average of more than $9,000 a year in New York City toward the cost of medical care received by those over sixty-five. For low-income persons and those who become indigent because of the cost of their care, the state spends an average of almost $19,000 per person. Most of these Medicaid dollars go for covering nursing home and home care costs not covered by the Medicare program. Family members also chip in to help cover the costs of this care and informally provide much of it themselves. Excluding savings and the sup-

Table 1.1 Resources for Paying for Care in New York City

	Total Persons 65 and Over[1]	Dollars per Person	Total Dollars
Income and Assets[2]			
Income	1,005,227	$25,205	$25.3 billion
Net Worth[3]	1,005,227	$311,000	$312.6 billion
Health Insurance			
Medicare[4]	846,364	$9,000	$7.6 billion
Medicaid[5]	254,083	$19,302	$4.9 billion

   1. Estimated (Claritas 1998).

   2. 1998 Bureau of Economic Analysis estimates, age corrected by Federal Reserve 1998 Survey of Consumer Finance (Kennickell et al. 2000).

   3. City estimates for households from the 1998 Federal Reserve Survey adjusted for age and household size (Kennickell et al. 2000).

   4. Compiled from Health Care Financing Administration (now the Centers for Medicare and Medicaid Services) county data files for Medicare elderly enrollment, July 1, 1998, and average adjusted per capita cost for 1998.

   5. Profile-FY98–99, New York City, All Aid Categories, Age 65 and Over, New York State Department of Health (www.health.state.ny.us/nysdoh/medstat/medicaid_profiles/99/demographic/99cal65.htm).

port of adult children and other family members, a total of $37,500 per elderly New York resident helps to cover their living expenses, personal care expenses, and medical costs. The city alone, excluding the suburban counties in its metropolitan area, represents an elder care market of almost forty billion dollars.

Paying for this care is complicated by two problems. The first is that paying for care blends funds for living expenses with health insurance payments. Pensions, Social Security, and SSI payments for the low-income elderly work differently than health insurance. Insurance typically pays for rare, unpredictable, catastrophic events. Insurance companies don't want to pay for services individuals want. That pits the interests of the individual against those of the insurance company and creates what insurance companies call a "moral hazard." Also, in order to make the insurance affordable, plans must limit what they will pay for and whom they will pay. Typically there are no similar constraints on what individuals can do with their own retirement income. However, for the elderly indigent, health insurance payments are usually more generous than those that cover their routine living expenses. For example, the New York State Medicaid Program pays nursing homes between $118 and $244 per person per day for care. In contrast, an adult home that cares for a person who only needs board, room, and personal care gets $27 per person per day. In calls to kennels in Manhattan, we found that this was half the typical cost per day for boarding a dog.

Care will be provided where the money is. Consequently, care will more often take place in health-related rather than social or residential settings. For example, according to actuarial adjustments used in computing Medicare-managed care rates in the United States in 2000, the "dually eligible" elderly, those who receive benefits from both Medicare and Medicaid, have hospital expenditures, correcting for age and sex differences, that are 1.7 times higher than those who receive only Medicare payments. The Medicare costs for physician services are 1.4 times higher for the dually eligible. In 1999, the elderly poor in the United States used 44% more hospital days than the nonpoor (National Center for Health Statistics 2001, 17). There is an inverse relationship between how much Medicare pays for hospital care and how much income individuals have. The average health expenditure (out-of-pocket and insurance-covered expenses) among elderly Medicare beneficiaries in the lowest income quintile was $12,602 in 1996. In the highest income quintile the average was $6,360, half as much (Forum on Aging-Related Statistics

2000). If all Medicare beneficiaries were as healthy and used health services as infrequently as the highest income quintile, $2,382 per person would be saved. That would be enough to cover a generous prescription and home care benefit package for everyone. Reflecting this same tendency, there is a direct relationship between neighborhood poverty and hospital use in New York City. Use rises with the degree of poverty in neighborhoods (Billings et al. 1993). Those who might have been more appropriately managed on an ambulatory basis are more likely to be admitted for inpatient care in low-income neighborhoods of New York City. For reasons I will make clear in the historical analysis in the next chapter, there is ample funding available for low-income individuals who need inpatient medical care but a paucity of resources for their daily living expenses.

The pooling of resources covering living and medical expenses is fraught with complications. For example, health insurance will pay for board and care in a hospital or a nursing home but not in one's own home. On the other hand, food stamps and Section 8 low-income rent subsidies can help support a person living independently but cannot be used to defray their cost in a health facility.

The blending of health care and day-to-day living in the same formal setting, as I will describe in detail in later chapters, also creates tensions between those providing and receiving care. Decisions about an individual's care go beyond the accounting problems of figuring out who should pay for what. Such decisions involve the problems of determining who is qualified to provide what kind of services and who decides what is purchased. An individual is free to decide what he will eat, where he will live, and whom he will hire to provide assistance in his own home. However, a physician (or maybe an insurance company) decides what medications patients should take, whether they should be hospitalized, and what care they should receive during hospitalization. What happens when health care and day-to-day living takes place in the same setting and one has to make decisions about how to allocate the same common pool of dollars? Who is in charge? These are not new conflicts, but when these different factors come into play in a common setting, they are certainly heightened.

As long as individuals pay for all of their care out of their own pockets, issues about who is in charge are clear. This is, however, the rare exception. Once individuals exhaust most of their income and assets, they can receive monthly SSI payments jointly administered by the federal government and the state. They can also become eligible for a variety of housing subsidies, food stamps, and Medicaid coverage of medical and some personal care expenses that are not covered by Medicare. Public dollars and charitable endowments also provide direct subsidies to providers of care to the indigent. Of course, as one moves from costs covered by one's own income and assets to costs covered as a beneficiary of an insurance plan to costs covered by direct charitable and public subsidies, control shifts from the recipient to the provider. One moves from a simple market transaction to a more complex set of relationships and expectations.

The second problem that makes paying for care more complicated is the inequitable distribution of income and assets. In 1998 New York's elderly population had an average income of $25,205 and an average net worth of $311,000. If all the elderly in New York were average, of course, the problems of providing and financing care for them would disappear, and this book would be unnecessary. Private housing and health services complexes target their developments to people with such income and wealth because they will usually have no difficulty paying for them. The problem is that no one is average. Income and assets are not equally distributed. Two thirds of New York's elderly households have incomes of less than $25,000, putting privately financed care out of reach. Nationally, income inequality has been increasing since 1967 (Masumura 1996; Jones and Weinberg 2000). For the over-sixty-five population, income inequalities have been significantly higher than the population as a whole but have been declining since 1967 (Rubin et al. 2000). Economic inequalities are greater in large urban centers such as New York City. New York State as a whole has the largest income gaps of any state. Those in the top fifth of households earned on the average 14.7 times more than those in the bottom fifth in 1998 (United Way of America 2000). Income inequalities in New York City are substantially larger in the over-sixty-five population than in the population as a whole. (Gini coefficients, the most commonly used measure of income inequality, were calculated from 1989 household income data from the U.S. Census. The Gini coefficient for over-sixty-five households in New York City was .549 and .468 for all age households. In contrast, the Gini index for the United States a whole for over-sixty-five households was .486 and .408 for all households.) These income inequalities, from the perspective of those providing care to the frail elderly in congregate settings, are a two-edged sword. On the one hand, the majority of elderly New Yorkers can't afford the cost of private congregate living arrangements. On the other hand, for many of those who can, such arrangements offer a poor substitute for the amenities, privacy, and services they can receive in their own home.

Exacerbating this problem further is how income disparities affect health. Poor health and the need for care are inversely related to income. For example, in the United States it costs the Medicare program more than twice as much to provide the same benefits for older persons who are poor than for those who are not poor. Populations that have higher per capita incomes tend to have better health. However, once certain income thresholds are passed, income inequality rather than per capita income better explains why some populations have longer life expectancies and lower health care costs than others. For example, in the United States higher income inequality in metropolitan areas is associated with higher mortality rates at all levels of income (Lynch et al. 1998). Some argue that such results are a consequence of the burdens placed on social networks and social cohesion by inequality (Wilkinson 1996; Auerbach and Krimgold 2001). If this is the case, certainly the frail elderly, with their greater dependence on such networks, are the most vulnerable. They are, in essence, the canaries in the coal mine. Growing inequality may be a slippery slope that we have all begun to slide down, eroding our ability to find common solutions. As one recent author on the topic observed:

> With high inequality, of income and of wealth, it becomes easy to know whether one is likely in the long run to be a net gainer or net loser, from public programs of family assistance, pension security and health care.... High inequality threatens the willingness to share at the same time that it concentrates resources in the hands least inclined to be willing. In this way ... inequality threatens the ability of a society to provide for the weak, the ill and the old. (Galbraith 1998)

This book tells the story of the struggle to reinvent care for the frail elderly in light of this drift into increasing inequality. This chapter has used New York City to illustrate how the existing system of care works and how it is changing. Two paths now diverge. We have, however, traveled this road many times. In order to understand the choices we face, we have to understand the history behind them. I will present this critical piece of the story in the next chapter.

2
A Brief History of Care

> To Europe she was America, to America she was the gateway of the earth. But to tell the story of New York would be to write the social history of the world.
> —H. G. Wells, *The War in the Air*

This chapter presents the history and the alternative paths that have been chosen in the past in caring for the frail elderly in New York City. This sector of the population needs assistance with the same activities of daily living (e.g., ambulation, feeding, dressing, bathing, etc.) now as they always have. Understanding how this care has been provided in the past makes the present-day conflicts more predictable. In telling the story of the social history of care for the frail elderly in New York City, or anywhere else, it helps to break it down into two separate stories, one about the predictable recurring tensions in how such care is organized and one about the more recent and less predictable disruptions that have profoundly changed the nature of that care.

The Recurring Themes

In part, the story about care for the frail elderly is one that involves three recurring conflicts over the nature of that care, conflicts over its purpose, its organization, and the role of government.

Purpose

Well into the twentieth century, public debate about how to care for the frail elderly was submerged in the debate about of how to deal with the poor. There was little that medicine could offer that could make any difference, and families informally provided most of the day-to-day care that was needed. The frail elderly represented only a tiny fraction of the population. In 1900 only one tenth of 1% of the population of the United States was over the age of eighty-five. In 2000 the proportion of the population over eighty-five had grown more than sixteenfold to 1.6% and was projected to reach 4.6%, or almost twenty million, by 2050 (Federal Interagency Forum on Aging-Related Statistics 2000, 56). The poor, however, of which the frail elderly represented only a small fraction, have always been a concern. The debate over how to handle the indigent has hinged on how much government should focus on attempting to eliminate, or at least ameliorate, the problems of poverty and how much just on controlling it. The prevailing position in New York City, as elsewhere in the United States, has been that attempts to alleviate poverty might well attract an even greater concentration of poor, and so efforts should focus on control. Throughout the city's four-hundred-year history, the fear that beggars, petty thieves, the homeless, and unruly mobs would inundate the city focused concern on policing the poor. Those fears helped shape care for the frail elderly.

Organization

A second related conflict involved whether to organize such care around "outdoor" or "indoor" relief. *Indoor relief* means providing care in an institution, an approach that is based on the assumption that residents and their care can be better controlled in such a setting. *Outdoor relief* means either providing financial support so that recipients can purchase what they need for themselves or directly providing food, fuel, and personal assistance in the recipients' own homes. These differing approaches raise the question, Should care be institutionalized or deinstitutionalized? How this question is answered reflects the perceived purpose of such care and the relationship between those providing the services and those receiving it. If those who are to receive care are considered dangerous or destructive to themselves or to the social fabric of a community, then it is likely that the community will choose to provide care through indoor relief. If the recipients of such care are seen as being like other members of communities, then the balance shifts toward the more sympathetic, more attractive, and less stigmatized treatment provided by outdoor relief (Lowell et al. 1900).

The conflict over indoor as opposed to outdoor relief, however, has also been a conflict over which costs less. The advantage of indoor relief is that the number of people receiving care through institutions can be restricted, and thus costs can be controlled. However, per recipient, outdoor relief is far cheaper. For example, in Massachusetts in 1889, the average cost of keeping a pauper in an almshouse was $180 per year, but the average cost for each "outdoor" pauper was only $40 per year (Lowell et al. 1900, 99). Thus, simply by shifting paupers from indoor to outdoor relief the cost could be reduced by more than 75%. In 1950 a similar conclusion was reached by the Municipal Hospital System in New York, which found that shifting hospital patients to its newly established home care program (e.g., outdoor relief) would not only relieve the overcrowding of the hospitals but would cost an average of only $2.66 per day, approximately one fourth the cost of general care on the wards of the municipal hospitals ("Home Care" 1950). In 1964, mayoral candidate John Lindsay argued for a dramatic expansion of nursing home beds on similar grounds, noting that the cost of care in the more institutionalized municipal hospital settings was $48 per day for each patient, but the cost would be only $15 per day for each patient in nursing homes (Lindsay 1964). While the costs of the services involved in computing such ratios have grown by a factor of more than ten, similar arguments are made today about the savings that could be obtained by shifting care from skilled nursing homes to home care or assisted living settings, and remarkably similar cost ratios are quoted.

Outdoor relief, however, is more attractive to the recipient and not limited by the physical capacity of a building. That makes controlling the costs and the number of recipients of such care more difficult. The fear has always been that outdoor relief would attract more recipients and end up costing far more. The concern is that outdoor benefits, rather than substituting for indoor care and thus saving money, would greatly expand costs by expanding use to those who might otherwise receive the same care informally from family members. Medicaid officials in many states today refer to this as the "woodwork problem." Pointing to New York State's experience in recent years, they argue that the expansion of benefits for home health services will increase the overall cost of long-term care for the Medicaid program.

Often, however, the choice between indoor and outdoor relief has had less to do with what is more cost-effective or consistent with prevailing beliefs than with the desire to shift costs to other parties. For example, when states assumed responsibility for the chronically mentally ill population at the end of the nineteenth century, local officials saw it as a golden opportunity to shift the cost of caring for the elderly in local almshouses to the state hospitals (Grob 1994, 548). Both the population and the average age of residents in state psychiatric hospitals grew dramatically in the first three decades of the twentieth century (Sutton 1991). This flow was reversed in the 1960s and 1970s, partly as a result of the opportunity that arose to shift the financial burden onto the federal government by moving the elderly psychiatric population to nursing homes and adult homes, where the costs of medical care would be reimbursable through the Medicare and Medicaid programs (Mechanic and Rochefort 1990).

Public Role

What should the role of government be in providing, financing, and regulating care for the frail elderly? Should it be a matter of limited public concern best left to the resources of individuals and their families? Is it just another good or service best left to the market, or is it part of a broader public responsibility to provide some level of security to citizens in old age? Such questions have risen to the surface only in the wake of periodic disclosures of financial abuses and substandard care that have sparked outrage.

Most of the time, the predominant view has been that government's role should be one of last resort, discouraging and controlling pauperism. Perhaps such periodic political outbursts over the conditions of care for the frail elderly are inevitable given the tensions over the purpose and organization of such care. In any event, these cycles of scandal, reform, and neglect are interwoven into the history of care in New York as they are across the nation as a whole.

The Case of New York

In New York City, recurring tensions over the purpose and role of government in the care of the frail elderly and over the organization of such care persisted through six successive periods.

A Focus on Relief for the Poor in the Dutch Settlement (1624–1664)

The original settlement in New York tended to focus on providing relief for the poor. Alleviation of conditions of the poor rather than control was the dominant theme during the Dutch West India Trading Company's occupation for three reasons. First, the Dutch poor relief system was probably the most advanced in Europe, and a focus on relief was taken for granted. The Dutch relief system of the time consisted of hospitals, workhouses, orphan asylums, and local almshouses where the aged could find shelter. The system was supported by widespread charity and public dollars (Schneider 1938, 9). Indeed, the Dutch continue to provide their citizens one of the best-developed and most comprehensive health and social welfare systems in the world. (As I will describe in the next chapter, a system similar to that of the Dutch recently returned and has indirectly influenced the dramatic growth of assisted living in the United States in the 1990s.) Second, the frontier environment required the people of all social classes to pull together to survive. Care for the frail elderly involved directly helping neighbors and was organized at the most natural local focal point, the church parish. Finally, during most of this period, the number of people needing relief and, as a result, their demands on resources were modest (Schneider 1938,15). The duty of providing for the welfare of the poor was entrusted to the clergy of the Dutch Reformed Church. Collections were taken up every Sunday and were occasionally supplemented by individual bequests or donations. It was also customary to provide a poor box at weddings to collect from guests. Local ordinances allocated a portion of fines to the poor fund. The first lottery was introduced in New Amsterdam in 1655 as a means of increasing the poor fund. Unlike its modern-day successors with their multimillion-dollar jackpots, all the winner of this lottery could expect to receive was a Bible (Schneider 1938, 14). Translating this experience to the present, a single standard of care for the frail elderly would become a reality if (1) it was consistent with the public's expectations, (2) the lives of the rich and poor were closely intertwined, and (3) the costs were relatively modest.

Relief provided during the Dutch settlement period reflected these conditions. It was provided to individuals in their own homes with neighborly familiarity and none of the stigma later associated with such assistance. Most of the assistance came in the form of food, fuel, and help with chores. Visitation of the sick and frail elderly was part of the duties of the Dutch Reformed ministry. This function was often entrusted to *sickentroosters* ("comforters of the sick"), who lacked the credentials of regularly ordained clergy. Such comforters of the sick or parish nurses have recently been rediscovered as a particularly cost-effective and more accepted way of supporting the frail elderly in their homes. A deacon's house, New Amsterdam's first poorhouse, was erected in 1653 (Schneider and Deutsch 1941, 12). It served only a small fraction of those receiving relief, but there was no stigma associated with residence in such houses as there would be in later years. Even those with the social eminence of clergy, lacking other arrangements, looked at such deacon's houses as welcome lodging (Schneider 1938,12). Although the Dutch West Indies settlement experienced many difficulties, caring for the poor was not one of them. It involved little in the way of resources, and the deacon's houses that were erected had few inmates. Indeed, deacons entrusted with the poor funds were accustomed to loaning out the surplus money at interest, accumulating reserves just as many modern health insurance plans do. There was a homey and neighborly character to the relief that local deacons provided with that money. Costs itemized in the account book of one deacon included payments for wet-nursing a child, a loan to a parishioner who pawned a pair of socks until his loan could be repaid, and funeral-related expenses associated with building a coffin, digging a grave, and providing brandy for the wake (Schneider 1938). (Jaded current providers of such services might be tempted to observe that the same resourceful deacon today would have risked newspaper exposé and a jail sentence for Medicaid fraud.)

Controlling the Poor in the British Colony (1664–1780)

Following the Dutch surrender of the New York colony to the British in 1664, laws and practices related to the poor in the colony shifted to reflect the different expectations and experiences of the new mother country. The new laws reflected a concern for controlling the movement of workers and the unemployed. An English law enacted in 1388 required those unable to work to be returned to the village of their birth. Those able to work but failing to do so would be subjected to a series of increasingly severe penalties, beginning with public whipping for the first offense, loss of ears for the second, and hanging for the third. A subsequent act prescribed the branding of vagabonds. With the enclosure of common fields for pastureland, many rural peasants were driven off the land. The Settlement Act of 1662 made it lawful to remove any newcomer on the suspicion that they might become a parish charge. The colony of New York followed suit with similar legislation in 1683. Skilled laborers were usually welcomed, but poor unskilled migrants were viewed with suspicion. Migrants who might prove a drain on the local community's poor funds were passed from local constable to local constable until they were returned to their place of origin. If such a person were to return to the place from which he or she had been removed, the person would be subject to being "stripped from the waist upwards and receiv[ing], if a man not exceeding thirty lashes and if a woman not exceeding twenty five lashes on the bare back and so as often as he or she shall return after such transportation" (Schneider 1938, 50).

For New York City, however, many immigrants bound for elsewhere had entered through the New York port. They were often returned there, and the municipality faced the dilemma of maintaining them indefinitely as public charges or absorbing the cost of returning them to their country of origin. For other municipalities, the cost of transportation was less expensive. As a result, New York City increasingly became a dumping ground for the outlying municipalities. The only colony-wide laws were those related to the "prevention" of indigence by preventing settlement. There were no uniform relief programs. Following similar requirements in England, a 1707 New York City Common Council decree required paupers to wear an "NY" mark in cloth on their person. Paupers were supported in their own homes or boarded with families. Increasingly, however, and particularly in New York City, those arrangements were inadequate to stem the growing problem of policing the poor.

The Elizabethan Poor Law of 1601, which served as the basic blueprint for general poor relief in Great Britain and its colonies, established a system of three different types of institutions for three distinct classes of paupers: (1) a poorhouse for those unable to work (e.g., the ill and the frail elderly), (2) a workhouse for those able to work but unable to find employment, and (3) a house of correction for the able-bodied who were unwilling to work (the unworthy poor). In practice, it was difficult to distinguish one class from another. For example, New York City completed the first public institution constructed to serve all three of these purposes in 1736. It was a two-story structure called the House of Correction, Workhouse and Poor House. The nomenclature for the building reflected city government's priorities. It was suitably furbished with fetters, shackles, and facilities for applying the lash. "Outpatient services" were supplied on a fee-for-service basis to slaveholders, who could send their slaves to the institution to be whipped. The westernmost division of the cellar of the building served for the confinement of the most unruly. A room on the west end of the upper floor was reserved for a six-bed infirmary. The infirmary would gradually expand, relocating several times and eventually becoming Bellevue Hospital. A new Bellevue almshouse was dedicated in 1816 on a twenty-six acre site along the East River. Although the three-story almshouse was the largest structure in the city, it was soon overflowing with people too young, old, or sick to offer any hope of being self-supporting. By 1825, the cost of its operation absorbed more than 10% of the city's budget. It housed as many as 1,867 inmates, almost one third of whom would die each year (Burrows and Wallace 1999, 503). The line between the almshouse inmates and an adjoining three-story stone penitentiary was blurred. Those who committed minor offenses, the vast majority guilty of vagrancy (which often meant nothing more than being unemployed, poor, and on the streets during occasional sweeps of the streets by city marshals at the behest of shopkeepers), were sentenced to the penitentiary and set to hard labor. When Bellevue Hospital was completed in 1826, the first two stories of the four-story structure were assigned to the insane poor. These public facilities would evolve into the city and county homes and farms of the early twentieth century and then into public nursing homes serving the Medicaid population. The stigma and ambivalence about improving conditions of care would persist.

Policing Eligibility for Relief in the New State (1780–1810)

As a result of the massive disruptions of the Revolutionary War, New York State for the first time participated directly in the provision of public relief. The war produced massive dislocations, including the exodus of more than three quarters of the population of New York City as a result of British occupation. Local responsibilities for relief that were assigned to church officials shifted to civil authorities. That shift placed the burden of caring for the poor on local governments, still reeling from the dislocations and impoverishment caused by the war. As a result, local authorities were increasingly concerned with controlling the cost of such care. As current state welfare and medical assistance program administrators well understand, there are two basic ways to control the cost of such programs: by restricting eligibility and by restricting services. They have followed the same path as their counterparts in the early years of the republic.

In order to assist the local municipalities with the increasing burden, New York State proceeded to reenact laws used in the colonial period to limit eligibility. The new laws focused on giving even smaller geographical units the responsibility for their own poor and established even more restrictive rules concerning eligibility. Those laws reinstated the procedures for passing on persons likely to become public charges from one constable to another to their place of origin as well as for whippings for those audacious enough to return.

The 1788 Poor Relief statute provided for the supervision in New York City of all forms of poor relief by the appointment of commissioners for the Almshouse and Bridwell (the combined jail and house of correction). The provision of relief had previously been the direct responsibility of Common Council. Its delegation to the supervisors of the almshouse and house of correction signaled the beginning of a fundamental shift in emphasis toward controlling cost by controlling services rather than eligibility.

Disciplining Workers in a Changing Economy (1810–1840)

For a variety of reasons still debated by historians, the Jacksonian Era began a shift toward addressing social problems by the construction of institutions (McEwen 1990). One major factor in the beginning of this trend was that the poor laws were increasingly at odds with the shift from an almost exclusively agrarian economy to the beginnings of an industrial one. The laws had to allow the flexibility for people to relocate in search of employment while still controlling local cost of poor relief. Pressures to reform poor relief in New York culminated in the legislature's commissioning a study of the problem by Secretary of State John Yates in 1823.

The Yates Report issued the following year included a comprehensive survey of poor relief in New York State, the first of its kind in the United States. Yates's survey of 367 towns found a total of 22,111 recipients of poor relief in a population of 1.5 million, or about 1.5% of the state's population. (By comparison, about 2.7 million people or 15% of New York State's population are currently eligible for Medicaid.) The recipients were divided into two classes, the "occasional" or "temporary" poor and the "permanent" poor. Of the 6,896 "permanent" poor, 928 were identified as aged and infirm. New York City alone accounted for about 42% of those receiving poor relief in the state and the highest percentage of residents on relief (7%). (In 1998 New York City accounted for about 65% of those eligible for Medicaid in the state, and about 24% of the city's population is Medicaid eligible.) The Yates survey classified the local methods of poor relief into four major categories: (1) "almshouse relief," (2) "home relief," (3) the "contract system" and (4) the "auction system." The "contract system" allowed for distributing those on poor relief to individuals who would be responsible for their supervision for a fixed rate per year. The contractor, usually a farmer, was granted the right to put his charges to work. More widespread than the contract system was the "auction system," which was the practice of auctioning off the poor to the person who would bid the lowest amount for the cost of their care. Its proponents felt that this approach, known as the "New England system" because of its widespread use in that region, had the added benefit discouraging individuals from applying for relief through the humiliation involved in standing for sale at a public auction. Its proponents argued the auction system also had another advantage. In many cases the low bidders themselves were on the edge of pauperism, desperate to avoid applying for relief themselves. Thus the town also benefited by being spared of having to provide that additional support. In some cases paupers were even auctioned off to their own relatives. In spite of the obvious potential for abuse, many towns were satisfied with the savings that these arrangements afforded them.

These four forms of relief persist in current arrangements in the United States in the form of nursing homes (almshouses), home care (home relief), and various forms of Medicaid- and Medicare-managed care and foster care (variations of the contract and auction systems). The contract system also evolved into the adult homes like those first operated by sometimes economically marginal individuals for the disabled and elderly indigent and more recently by publicly traded national corporations for the private market. The Yates Report criticized the existing relief system, arguing that the battles over settlement and removal were a costly waste of scarce resources and often cruel to the recipients of relief; that the contract and auction system was barbaric; and that with the exception of the almshouse arrangements, all failed to encourage more productive habits. The study recommended the elimination of the orders of removal and a shift to the exclusive use of indoor or almshouse relief. Watered-down legislation embodying these two recommendations passed the following year. It represented a fundamental shift in policy and reflected the beginning of the transformation from an agrarian economy to an industrial one, which required greater labor mobility. As a result of the change, the lifeline that was based on a sense of responsibility for the poor and frail elderly within a community was severed. Costs would now be controlled by the new discipline and direction promised by indoor relief by controlling the services offered to relief recipients.

The reformers believed that indoor relief would not only provide for the maintenance of paupers but would cure the fundamental cause of pauperism. As argued in the Yates Report, inadequate supervision of relief recipients contributed to pauperism, as "a great proportion of the paupers are voluntary, a consequence of drunkenness, idleness and vice of all kinds." The object of indoor relief was to make gainful employment of any kind a far more desirable option. As has often been the case since, the simplistic assumptions in the arguments of the reformers bore little resemblance to the more complex and harsher realities.

Saving Children and the Mentally Ill from the Almshouses (1840–1890)

The shift to indoor relief, the almshouse approach, as the dominant form of relief eventually forced a more careful assessment of almshouse residents that challenged the simplistic moralistic assumptions about the causes of their plight. Many groups organized to rescue children and the mentally ill from such a cruel and unfair fate. Voluntary groups formed to create private institutions as an alternative for the more "deserving poor." Most of the voluntary hospitals in New York had their origins from such efforts. Those with drug and alcohol problems, sexually transmitted diseases, and criminal records were unlikely to be defined as deserving of such private charity. Many of the ethnic groups established charitable hospitals and homes to care for their "own kind" whose plight could motivate charitable giving. Meanwhile, reformers in the last half of the nineteenth century succeeded in removing from the almshouse various subgroups of "deserving" poor and placing them in settings more appropriate to assuring their welfare.

As they often have since, children served as the first and easiest target. The New York Association for Improving Conditions of the Poor was organized in 1843. It focused on addressing the needs of vagrant and neglected children. The association's efforts bore fruit with the establishment of the New York Juvenile Asylum in 1851. Meanwhile, the

Children's Aid Society, founded in 1853, worked to improve the conditions for children in almshouses. The population of children in poorhouses throughout the state, however, increased fourfold during the Civil War years. Efforts to improve conditions soon gave way to a movement to remove children from almshouses altogether. These efforts culminated in the passage of the Children's Act of 1875, which prohibited keeping children between the ages of three and sixteen in almshouses.

The mentally ill were another target of reform groups. The governor appointed a committee of inquiry to investigate the conditions of the insane, which submitted its report in 1831. As a consequence, the first state lunatic asylum was finally opened in 1843 in Utica. In one of her state surveys, which would transform the treatment of the mentally ill throughout the nation, Dorothea Dix urged the removal of the insane from poorhouses and jails to special institutions for care and treatment. She argued that they were wards of the state and not the financial responsibility of local municipalities. It would take almost fifty years to make the shift of financial burden a reality. Only acute cases were accepted at the state facility at Utica. Chronic cases remained in the local jails and almshouses. In 1855 Dr. Sylvester Willard conducted a statewide inquiry confirming the shocking conditions of neglect and brutality previously reported by Dix and others. The state legislature established the Willard State Asylum for the Chronic Insane in 1865. It was the largest state mental institution in the country. With the addition of this institution and others that would follow over the next fifty years, New York State relocated all of the insane from county facilities to the state acute or chronic asylums.

Nothing, however, would have changed without the efforts of such influential advocacy groups as the State Charities Aid Association. The State Charities Aid Association served as the model for many advocacy groups that would follow, including the Nursing Home Community Coalition of New York State, which assisted in the completion of this book. Formed in 1872, the State Charities Aid Association proceeded to develop visiting committees in almost every county in the state. With the support of the state Commissions of Public Charities, the state Supreme Court in 1881 granted the association the right to inspect any almshouse in the state. The association served as the major force behind welfare changes until the Old Age Security Act was enacted in 1930. Its survey of the county facilities in 1883 revealed little progress in addressing the needs of the mentally ill. They noted:

If special quarters in poorhouses are assigned to the insane, they are often in those parts of the building least useful for other purposes, in attics and basements, and often in outbuildings. The insane mingle with other paupers and whatever may have been their antecedents, they are often condemned to association with the idiotic and the intemperate—those who are morally and mentally degraded. They are left filthy and squalid; they lounge about idle, in shadeless yards made offensive by neglected privies; there is little effort to keep the sexes apart, and no regular attempt to cure the patients or even to improve their condition. Statistics furnished to the public by the State Commissioner of Lunacy show that a majority of the insane in county asylums and poorhouses have never had anything better than poorhouse custody. They have never been treated in State hospitals, and therefore presumably have never had the chance for recovery due them. Taken to the poorhouse at the outset, they have remained in the poorhouse and made chronic cases by county neglect. (quoted in Schneider and Deutsch 1941, 92–93)

Finally, in 1890, the State Care Act directed that all insane in county institutions be moved as rapidly as accommodation could be afforded them to state hospitals, where the state alone would bear all of the expense for their care.

During the fifty-year struggle to transfer the mentally ill to state care, many other specialized state facilities had been created to meet the special needs of the mentally handicapped, the blind, and the deaf, who had traditionally been housed in the almshouses. The only major almshouse population untouched by these nineteenth-century reforms was the impoverished elderly.

Saving the Elderly from the Almshouses (1890–1929)

By 1920 the transformation of the almshouse as an institution mainly for the care of the aged and infirm was complete (Schneider and Deutsch 1941). Roughly 1% of the population over sixty-five years of age in the United States was housed either in local public facilities or their voluntary counterparts. The poorhouse was defined as a consequence of the failure to provide adequate old-age pensions. Proposals for old age pension plans were played off against exposés concerning conditions in the almshouses. Harry C. Evans's 1926 study *The American Poorfarm and Its Inmates,* based on a survey supported by several fraternal organizations, described shocking conditions in New York and other states. A less inflammatory study by the National Civic Federation came to similar conclusions. It described a crowded, depressing environment in one New York facility:

> The almshouse buildings on Welfare Island typify the institutional architecture of a century ago, differing little either in construction or atmosphere from their neighboring penal buildings. Adapting them to a new era and more enlightened standard of indigent care is extremely difficult, perhaps impossible.
>
> The men's quarters are seriously overcrowded and the basement of the Catholic Church has been converted into a dormitory, housing 200 men. The building occupied by blind men is dilapidated and probably unsafe for the type of patients it houses. The recreation hall is a dismal, barn-like place furnished with long wooden benches and used as a lounging, smoking and day room by the men. The women's sitting room is a long, narrow room, crowded and disorderly. (quoted in Schneider and Deutsch 1941, 281)

The New York legislature appointed its own joint committee to investigate conditions in 1926. The report of the legislature was based on inspections of almost all the public almshouses in the state. The report stated:

> At least two of the older institutions in the State were formerly insane asylums. The tall, narrow barred windows and the iron-barred doors on the old cells give anything but a homelike atmosphere. . . . Some of the older buildings have narrow, dark rickety stairways, which are dangerous. Some of the older institutions are sadly deficient in heating equipment. Probably, the greatest shortcomings of institutions of today are the lack of hospital facilities. . . . [T]here is practically no provision made for any occupations to take up the inmates' time. (quoted in Schneider and Deutsch 1941, 281)

The final recommendation of the report was that an unbiased investigation should be made of retirement and old-age pension plans.

The 1929 Public Welfare Act was the culmination of efforts of reformers to legislate change. The law reversed the principle of the 1824 County Poorhouse Act. It stated that "wherever practical relief shall be given to the poor person in his own home" (quoted in Thomas 1969, 30). The reformers had been arguing since early in the century that an adequate pension system would eliminate the need for the shameful blight and public cost of almshouses. More careful study of the elderly inmates had shown that few were physically and mentally able to care for themselves (Hoffman 1908, 188). Such facts were ignored in the advocacy of pension legislation, which created much subsequent mischief. In 1929 the legislature also created the Commission on Old Age Security. That commission's report led to the enactment of the state's Old Age Security Act of 1930, which restricted such assistance to the poor to those who were not in institutions. Would the act serve to end punitive control and institutionalized confinement of the indigent frail elderly, or would demands for public action to control abuse continue?

Change

I have used the story up until 1930 to illustrate the unresolved conflicts over the purpose, organization, and importance of public involvement in care for the frail elderly. Long-term care in the United States continues to be shaped by these recurring conflicts. Most state Medicaid programs provide limited home health benefits and invest the vast majority of funds in nursing home care, or "indoor" relief, using arguments similar to their nineteenth-century counterparts. Nursing homes retain the stigma of their nineteenth-century predecessors, and most elderly persons view them more as a dreaded form of imprisonment than as a place of refuge. Unlike other forms of health care, nursing home care is not provided for by any public or private insurance coverage of any significance. Nursing homes are places where most people are either admitted as indigents or, if they live long enough, become indigents. Efforts at reinventing care have tried to offer alternatives.

Things do change, however. Unanticipated disturbances disrupted these old patterns after 1930. Three waves of change profoundly affected care to the frail elderly: the Great Depression of the 1930s, the social movements of the 1960s, and the economic transformation of the 1990s. Each produced a sequence of three shock waves: a major disruption in society that shattered existing arrangements of care, an effort to change the care system to address the effects of the disruption, and a sequence of aftershocks produced by the unintended consequences of these changes. However, the story is more complex. The disruptions had a cumulative effect that resulted in even more profound changes in the organization of health and social services as a whole and in society in general. While the account that follows focuses on what happened in New York, it mirrors almost identical events in other states and in the nation as a whole.

Aftershocks of the Great Depression: Destruction of the Almshouses and Emergence of the Proprietary Nursing Home (1930–1960)

The Great Depression in the 1930s shook existing patterns of care for the frail elderly. The existing system of support based on local responsibility and a patchwork of nonprofit charitable and public facilities collapsed when the tidal wave of need caused by the Depression engulfed it. Outdoor relief, or providing direct payments to recipients rather than committing them to institutions, gained broad support when it became clear that both the stigma and practicality of indoor relief no longer made sense. With the election of Franklin Delano Roosevelt as president, New York's own Old Age Security legislation became incorporated into the pending national Social Security legislation. Reflecting the original New York law and the legacy of exposés on the almshouses, the proposed federal legislation disallowed aid to persons who were "inmates of public or other charitable institutions" (Thomas 1969, 49). Quick to defend the financial interests of their members, the voluntary hospital associations objected. The final bill excluded payment only to inmates of public institutions. Those crafting and supporting the legislation promoted it as honorable public support for those who deserved it. That stance was in stark contrast to the stigmatized relief and abysmal poorhouse conditions of the past. Thus the Social Security Act of 1935 redefined the relationship between citizens and the federal government. The role of government in the care of the frail elderly was no longer viewed as a local police function.

The Social Security Act's measures to discourage indoor relief, however, unintentionally stimulated its resurgence in new forms. Local welfare administrators, who were denied a federal subsidy to support inmates in county and municipal facilities, shifted them to private boarding homes, where the new Old Age Assistance payments reduced local government's financial burden. Private for-profit boarding homes opened to fill an increasing need for places to send Old Age Assistance recipients. However, since elderly persons now had "outdoor" relief in the form of Old Age Assistance and Social Security, only those who were physically unable to live independently continued to live in these homes. The residents in the private boarding homes became older, sicker, and increasingly more frail. Many of the private boarding homes responded to the growing needs of their residents and transformed themselves into nursing homes. By the 1950s, for-profit facilities had emerged as the dominant form of nursing home ownership in the United States.

As elsewhere, the emergence of a for-profit nursing home sector in New York State filled a void left by the private charitable facilities. The upstate charitable homes restricted admission to individuals in reasonable health and members of their own religious faith or fraternal order. Some refused to accept persons on assistance. Waiting lists at such charitable facilities enabled a good deal of selectivity in terms of who was admitted. The majority of the homes required admission fees that were not covered by public assistance programs.

Yet the real stumbling block that prevented the private charitable institutions from serving the indigent was cultural. As private organizations, they did not want to become embroiled in government procedures and regulations that admission of public charges would entail. It also didn't help that local welfare administrators usually tried to take advantage of the charitable nature of those institutions that were willing to work with them by paying them far less than the full cost of the care they provided (Thomas 1969, 68).

Most of the early for-profit operators were similar to those who had contracted with local municipalities or bid for the care of paupers at public auctions in the early part of the nineteenth century. As one commentator observed, they "seem typically to have begun when women with invalid husbands took in other invalids for fees to help pay the bills" (Thomas 1969, 74). It was a way for those who had a home but were unemployed and those with marginal residential real estate holdings to make at least a meager living, but it was hardly a promising formula for assuring adequate care for residents. Boarding home fires and scandals related to mistreatment and abuse of residents were frequent in the 1940s and 1950s. The average size of the upstate facilities had grown to only fourteen beds by 1949.

The growth of proprietary nursing homes in New York City lagged behind their development upstate because those in the city were constrained by municipal regulation. The city Department of Hospitals, created in 1929, had responsibility for inspecting and licensing nursing homes. Licenses had to be renewed each year, and the operation of an unlicensed facility was punishable by a fine and up to a year in prison. The code required, among other things, that registered nurses be in charge of the nursing and custodial care of patients, that there be at least one toilet per eight patients, and that buildings more than twenty feet in height be of fireproof construction. State regulation of proprietary homes upstate did not begin until 1951.

Unlike the upstate homes, proprietary homes in New York City provided care in an environment that was dominated by large municipal hospitals and charitable homes for the aged. A census conducted in 1928 revealed that many frail elderly were cared for in the beds of the twenty general and specialty hospitals in the municipal system (Jarrett 1933, 1:240–41). In addition, two municipal facilities, the City Home and the Farm Colony, both of which were direct descendents of the city's almshouse, provided care specifically for New York's indigent frail elderly population. The City Home, which was located on Welfare Island (now Roosevelt Island), provided care for 1,717 predominantly elderly residents. Its physical layout, essentially unchanged from the almshouse located there in 1847, included two large stone barracks, one housing men and the other women. The other city institution, the Farm Colony on Staten Island, included mostly similar barracks that could house a population of about 1,200. In a marked departure from its historical roots and as a demonstration of what is possible in providing privacy and amenities to residents in a public institution, the Farm Colony included two thirty-unit "cottages," with private rooms, separate kitchens, and sitting and dining rooms. At the time, before the Great Depression scuttled hopes of their realization, plans were in place to expand the "Cottage Colony" to fourteen cottages on its forty-acre site. The planning of those cottages anticipated by more than fifty years the private assisted living communities that developed in the 1990s (Jarrett 1933, 2:250). In general, however, conditions for the chronically ill were abysmal in the city, as noted in a 1928 survey:

> The inmates are crowded into antiquated buildings with inadequate occupational and recreational facilities. The most flagrant defects are the tremendous crowding of the wards and the utter lack of privacy for the inmates. No locker space whatsoever is provided for personal belongings. The sitting rooms on the invalid wards are too small; the toilets and lavatories are too few in number. The recreation hall, which serves as a sitting room for all of the ambulant patients, is much too small. The dining room is dark, dismal, and crowded. The food is served hot, but the method of service and the metal dishes used are very unappetizing. (quoted in Jarrett 1933, 1:251–52)

In addition, the 1928 New York City census identified a large nonprofit sector serving the frail elderly, which included 87 homes for the aged, which housed 8,343 residents (Jarrett 1933, 2:126). Like their upstate counterparts, most of these homes attempted to restrict admission to the able-bodied aged. Nevertheless, almost half their occupants were chronically ill, and 10% were bedridden (Jarrett 1933, 101). All but ten of these homes excluded blacks, and four of those were operated for blacks only (Jarrett 1933, 2:125–26). Forty-five of the eighty-seven homes restricted admission based on religious creed. Thirty-one required admission fees ranging from $100 to $5,000, thus excluding indigent applicants. While on the whole providing care in less congested and more attractive surroundings than the public homes, only nine of the homes provided exclusively single-room accommodations. Thirty-one provided at least some dormitory or ward accommodations for residents.

In addition to operating in the shadow of the nonprofits and municipal facilities, the private nursing homes were under the jurisdiction of the city Department of Hospitals, which conducted a persistent effort to close down marginal, physician-owned, for-profit hospitals in the city. Physicians unable to obtain privileges at the voluntary hospitals in the city operated many of the private hospitals. In 1940 there were as many as sixty-five for-profit hospitals in New York City, averaging about sixty beds each ("Private Hospital Loses" 1940). Essentially, the city Department of Hospitals had successfully closed down all but a handful of these for-profit hospitals by the end of the 1960s.

Nevertheless, the proprietary nursing homes were able to carve out a niche. That came about because the voluntary homes for the aged were unwilling to accept convalescent patients, and city officials saw the need for facilities that provided post-acute short-stay nursing care to reduce the pressure of high occupancy levels in the city's hospitals. While upstate proprietary nursing homes tended to concentrate on indigent cases, the city's proprietary nursing homes tended to be predominantly private pay. The city's regulators envisioned that the proprietary nursing homes would be restricted to providing places for post-hospital or convalescent care of no more than three months duration and not as places providing permanent living arrangements for the frail elderly. They restricted their growth accordingly. Inadvertently, however, they greatly strengthened the bargaining position of the proprietary nursing home operators. The city faced increasingly crowded conditions in the municipal hospitals after World War II. By 1950 beds were being squeezed into hallways, and the average occupancy rate in the municipal hospital system was over 100%. The highest was over 119% (Thomas 1969, 186). Adding to the pressure, the 1950 Social Security Amendments provided for a new reimbursable welfare category, "aid to the disabled," which further encouraged shifting patients from the municipal hospitals to nursing homes and shifting the cost onto the federal government. This resulted in an explosive growth of the proprietary nursing homes in the 1950s. They grew from 44 facilities with 884 beds and an average size of 20 beds in the early 1940s to 107 facilities with 9,420 beds and an average size of 88 beds by 1961 (Thomas 1969, 258).

Yet this temporary marriage of convenience did nothing to change the underlying hostility of the city and voluntary sector leaders toward the proprietary nursing homes. In 1958 the New York City commissioner on investigations, Louis I. Kaplan, began a two-year probe of the proprietary nursing homes in the city. On April 6, 1960, Kaplan submitted his report to Mayor Wagner. It was an angry indictment of the proprietary nursing home industry and the small group of operators who appeared to control it. As summarized in a later state commission report, the report concluded:

> Many operators were attracted purely by the opportunity to make substantial returns on capital investments and were neither socially motivated nor professionally equipped for the undertaking.
>
> 1. Public regulation . . . because of the profit incentive . . . had to become more vigorous if the public interest was to be served.
> 2. Proprietary nursing homes were inadequately staffed and were not qualified to carry out their responsibilities; the Department of Welfare and the Department of Hospitals had not assured the well being of patients by enforcing code requirements.
> 3. Nursing homes filed attendance records that had been deliberately falsified to assure licensure from the Department of Hospitals and appropriate classification for referrals from the Department of Welfare.
> 4. Nursing homes failed to give patients the care they contracted with the Department of Welfare to provide and thus overcharged the Department and City of New York.
> 5. Proprietary nursing homes were controlled by a cartel of promoters concerned only with profit.
> 6. One owner who never held a license in any of his homes controlled twenty-five homes. . . . [F]inancial investments were recorded in the names of friends and relatives.

7. Nursing home operators had committed crimes by filing false reports and false instruments. Many freely admitted to Kaplan's investigators that they had committed such crimes. "Just about every one admitted to filing false documents," said one of the investigators.
8. Between July 1, 1956, and June 30, 1958, these operators had overcharged the city $3.7 million.

> Kaplan recommended that (i) the city take steps to collect these overcharges and not increase payment to operators until the money had been recouped and (ii) the report be forwarded to the New York County District Attorney's office so that criminal prosecutions could be initiated. (Temporary State Commission 1975, 132–34)

A 1962 follow-up report found that there had been no improvement in the operation of the nursing homes and only a small fraction of the overcharges had been recouped.

The criticism of proprietary nursing homes, however, went well beyond issues of substandard care and fraud. Many medical leaders, both in the city and nationally, questioned the growing separation between nursing homes and the mainstream of medical care. In the preface to William Thomas's 1969 book on nursing home policy in the previous decades in New York, Martin Cherkasky, administrator of Montefiore Hospital, an early developer of hospital organized home health care and an advocate for the integration of the public and voluntary hospitals in the city, concluded that the proprietary nursing homes

> [a]ll too often . . . have been a disgrace to our society. The oldest, most pitiable, most helpless persons have been left to linger without hope in these institutions; most of their care and services have been poor; rehabilitative therapy has been nonexistent; and the physical surroundings and ambiance have been unappetizing and deadening. This is because nursing home care for the most part has been outside the mainstream of modern medicine. . . . [I]t is questionable whether such a crucial service should be substantially in the hands of entrepreneurs who frequently make large sums of money from the operation of these institutions. (Thomas 1969, viii–ix)

In spite of the concerns raised about an increasingly segregated nursing home sector and the role of for-profit ownership, those issues disappeared from the radar screen for more than a decade. Subsequent events accelerated the shift toward even more segregated care and increased dominance of for-profit ownership.

Aftershocks of the Civil Rights Movement:
The Effects of Medicare and Medicaid (1960–1990)

The second disturbance in the twentieth century that shattered existing patterns of care for the frail elderly began with the Civil Rights movement at the end of the 1950s. Its growing momentum helped tip the balance that enabled the passage of the Medicare and Medicaid legislation in 1965 (Smith 1999). In signing the bill in into law, President Johnson said:

> No longer will older Americans be denied the healing miracle of modern medicine. No longer will illness crush and destroy the savings they have so carefully put away over a lifetime so they might enjoy dignity in their later years. No longer will young families see their own income, and their own hopes eaten away simply because they are carrying out their deep moral obligations to their parents.... No longer will this Nation refuse the hand of justice to those who have given a lifetime of service and wisdom and labor to the progress of this progressive country. (quoted in De Lew 2000, 1)

The percentage of the federal budget that went to health care jumped from 10.9% in 1960 to 24.3% in 1970 (Health Care Financing Administration 1997a). This dramatic increase in federal spending on health care produced four interrelated, unanticipated, and seemingly contradictory changes in the care of the frail elderly: long-term care became increasingly segregated from short-term or acute care, long-term care became increasingly medicalized, psychiatric care became increasingly deinstitutionalized, and health care in general increasingly became a venture of private, for-profit corporations.

SEGREGATION OF LONG-TERM AND SHORT-TERM CARE

Long-term care became more separated from the acute care sector. In part, that separation was caused by the use of the Medicare program to pay the hospital costs of the elderly and the use of the Medicaid program to pay nursing home costs. The separation also reflected resistance to racial integration of long-term care services (Smith 1999). As a result, long-term care remained, as it had been for more than a century, part of state and local governments' responsibility for the poor and was separated from acute hospital care.

Federal dollars flowing through state Medicaid programs to nursing homes, however, stimulated dramatic growth. National expenditures for nursing home care jumped from $800 million to $4.2 billion during the 1960s, the bulk of this increase coming from state Medicaid funds. Expenditures for nursing home care grew at an average annual rate of 17.4% during the decade. Nursing home bed capacity in the United States more than doubled between 1963 and 1973, expanding to 1,174,900 and exceeding the bed capacity in acute care hospitals (National Center for Health Statistics 1975, 10). What emerged was an almost completely separate system of care, unlike what exists in any other developed country in the world. In other developed countries most so-called acute or short-term hospitals either directly provide or have administrative responsibility over an array of long-term care facilities and services.

AN INCREASED MEDICALIZATION OF CARE

The separation of long-term and short-term care, which might have been justified if it had been used to preserve a more social or noninstitutional model of care, coincided with an acceleration of more institutional and medicalized arrangements to care for the frail elderly. Just as the financial impact of Medicare and Medicaid helped bring about an increased separation of long-term care from short-term care, it also influenced a shift in the long-term care sector toward a more medical model of care. Medicare and Medicaid, unlike the original Social Security legislation, were not designed as programs to provide social or income support but as health insurance programs. Health insurance programs do two things to control the risks and the costs of their plans. First, benefits are not distributed to everyone enrolled in the plan but only to those experiencing losses. Second, health insurance restricts the recovery of such costs to only a narrow band of "qualified" providers. The costs of informal caregivers, alternative medicines, and those perceived to be "cultists" are not covered. Only the costs of acceptably licensed and credentialed providers are reimbursable, and then only if those costs reflect narrowly defined eligible services. Medicare and most state Medicaid programs, just like other health insurance plans, do not pay for help with household chores, ambulation, feeding, and so forth. Facilities that are not licensed as medical facilities (e.g., foster homes, boarding homes, and retirement condominiums) are not supported by those programs. Those defined as medical facilities, however, were generously compensated by Medicare and Medicaid for providing care to those with "real" medical needs. Not surprisingly, this produced dramatic growth in the number of skilled nursing home facilities that could take advantage of this generosity. It also produced a simultaneous effort by Medicare and Medicaid administrators to impose greater restrictions on such eligibility, in part to improve the quality of the programs but mostly in a largely futile attempt to control their costs.

Thus the massive growth in the number of nursing home beds tells only part of the story of the effect Medicare and Medicaid had long-term care. At the beginning of the 1960s, many proprietary nursing homes were wood-frame conversions of private homes. The average size of proprietary homes in 1963 was 25.9 beds. At least half of the nursing home beds that existed in the 1960s were in facilities that have since closed. The great growth in nursing home bed capacity resulted primarily from the opening of new facilities. New construction of nursing homes between 1965 and 1975 included approximately one million nursing home beds. The character of what was then described as the nursing home "industry" had changed dramatically. Chains, some national in scope, operated an increasing share of these homes. The greater standardization and predictability imposed by federal regulation of payment and care created the potential for real economies of scale that had not been possible before through locally administered programs.

Perhaps most significantly, however, the changes accompanied a dramatic shift in the character of the care provided in these homes. The homes became more medicalized, treating sicker patients. Nursing homes that had previously served as part of the welfare system became, increasingly, an extension of the health care system. Many of the older ma-and-pa operations were closed as a result. In New York State, for example, 291 of the 339 homes that closed between 1967 and 1974 had fewer than 50 beds each, and 251 of those smaller homes were proprietary. Most of these smaller, owner-operated homes could not meet the stricter building code standards now imposed on all medical facilities. An operator of one of these smaller homes that closed wrote the following protest letter to the editor of a local newspaper:

> What are you doing New Year's Eve? Would you and all the residents of Monroe County like to cancel your previous plans and join the nonconforming nursing homes in Monroe County? There won't be any liquor, balloons, or an orchestra, but there will be dancing. The dancer will be the geriatric patient, who is literally being pushed out on the street by New York State.
>
> You see we aren't built right. We aren't fire-resistant—but check out

with the fire departments as to how often they have answered a fire call to one of us. Our hallways aren't eight feet wide but more love and compassion travel down our narrow pathways than any 8–10 foot one. Ours expand with all the tender loving care one could desire and need, not by a carpenter's tool. (quoted in Smith 1981, 23)

The small, non-code-compliant, owner-operated homes in New York closed, in spite of protests, as they did elsewhere. They were replaced by larger, more medically oriented and more institutional facilities. Even the operators of the nursing homes that survived, who clearly benefited both professionally and financially from the changes, were ambivalent about them:

A group of nursing home operators at a conference were asked to describe their own facilities. Some described brand new facilities with elaborate recreational and physical therapy programs and over 300 beds. One facility was a thirty-bed operation run by a religious order. The home had a garden, some chickens, and a stream for fishing. The Sisters spoke with great affection and interest about each of their residents. At the end of the session the participants were asked to vote for the homes in which they would prefer to be a patient. The thirty-bed home of the Sisters was the unanimous choice! (Smith 1981, 154)

In the first decade after the passage of Medicare, a new, more impersonal set of institutions emerged. Organizationally separated from acute hospitals and from the welfare system, these institutions exceeded general hospitals in bed capacity. Nationally in fiscal year 1995 the Medicaid program paid more than $27 billion to nursing homes, more than it expended for inpatient care in acute hospitals, and public funds accounted for more than 58% of all nursing home revenue in 1995 (Health Care Financing Administration 1997b, Table 10).

No one could make much sense of the long-term care system that was emerging. In 1975 the Senate Special Committee on Aging published a report, *Doctors in Nursing Homes: The Shunned Responsibility*, bemoaning the medical neglect in the long-term care system. For every 1,000 nursing home beds in the United States, there were 250 costly transfers to hospitals, five times the rate of Great Britain's more integrated system (Barker 1987, 119). A position paper from the American College of Physicians' Health and Public Policy Subcommittee on Aging surveyed the barren landscape in 1984 and found:

At present, there is not a comprehensive system of long-term care for the elderly in the United States. A confusing, fragmented, and expensive system exists that contains both gaps and duplication of services. Consequently, many elderly do not receive the services they need, while others receive services inappropriately.... Reimbursement procedures, both public and private, tacitly recognize the existence of two separate systems of health care: one for acute care and another for long-term care. Such a division is unrealistic and results often in inadequate responses to the medical needs of the elderly. (American College of Physicians 1984, 763)

DEINSTITUTIONALIZATION OF THE PSYCHIATRIC HOSPITAL POPULATION

Adding to the difficulties of this newly emerging long-term care system was the effect of the Medicare and Medicaid programs on the state psychiatric hospital population. The Medicare and Medicaid programs, born out of pressures from the Civil Rights movement, provided not only a financial incentive for states to shift residents out of public institutionalized settings but also an ideology to support that shift. That ideology equated deinstitutionalization of the mentally ill and handicapped with equal rights. It signaled a major watershed in use of inpatient care in the United States. "We demand the total abolition of psychiatric institutions, since the function they serve is to imprison, torture and dehumanize people and not to help them," argued one national patient advocacy group in 1976 (Madness Network News 1976, 1). It is remarkable how close advocates came to getting what they wished for. It is also perhaps an object lesson on why one should be careful of what one wishes. The number of nonfederal public psychiatric beds dropped from 413,878 in 1970 to 63,525 in 1998 (Manderscheid et al. 2002, Table 2). In 1955 New York State's psychiatric hospitals had 93,314 patients, but by the year 2000 that number had dwindled to 4,850. While some of the patients who were moved out of the state psychiatric hospitals were absorbed into nursing homes, most were absorbed into single-room occupancy hotels and adult boarding homes. The results were often disastrous. A report by the Human Resources Administration in 1980 estimated that more than forty thousand state psychiatric patients had been released in New York City in the previous four years and that as many as ten thousand of them were currently living in single-room occupancy hotels in the city. Homeless shelters and the streets handled the growing overflow (Kihss 1980). To absorb some of the backlog, New York's municipal hospitals began to admit some of the patients. There was an average waiting time of 116 days for more appropriate placement at Kings County Hospital (Kihss 1982). The number of psychiatric hospital discharges among the residents in the adult homes across the state had grown to more than nine thousand by 1990. The Commission on Quality of Care for the Mentally Disabled, which made surprise inspections in forty-seven adult homes in 1990, found "conditions in the homes so wretched that they looked like the old back wards of mental hospitals of a generation ago" (Raab 1990). The larger homes and those in New York City tended to be the worst. More than a dozen residents of adult homes in the New York City area informed the commission investigators that employees routinely used the threat of eviction to prevent them from complaining to state inspectors about abuses, which included muggings by intruders, unsanitary conditions, lack of heat in the winter, and poor food (Raab 1990). The untold part of the story, repeated many times by adult home operators whom I interviewed, was the disruptive and often frightening impact that the younger psychiatric patients had on the frail, elderly long-term residents in some of the adult homes.

EMERGENCE OF THE CORPORATE PROVISION OF CARE

The final and perhaps most predictable consequence of the growth of the long-term care sector was the growing dominance of publicly traded corporations. The corporations established chains of nursing homes in the 1960s and early 1970s in response to the massive infusion of dollars from the Medicare and Medicaid programs. One of the early publicly traded nursing home chains was Medic Home Enterprises, which made its initial public offering of stock in 1968. Bernard Bergman served as an officer and was a major stockholder in Medic Home Enterprises. Through his wife, he also owned the Towers Nursing Home in Manhattan (Mendelson 1974, 104–8). A complex interconnected network of real estate ownership, which were operations described by investigative reporters and prosecutors as "the syndicate," involved Bergman in a multistate nursing home empire. Bergman had been a key unnamed party in the Kaplan investigation of overcharging and substandard care in the city's proprietary nursing homes. A turbulent sequence of events followed, resulting in a year of imprisonment for Bergman, restitution of money Bergman's facilities had fraudulently received from the Medicaid program, and the closing or transfer of ownership of most of Bergman's nursing home holdings in New York. It cast a shadow on publicly traded nursing home companies that persists to the present.

In New York City the concerns about the increasing for-profit ownership that had lain dormant resurfaced in 1974. Mirroring the Watergate exposé of the time, the *New York Times* and the *Village Voice* published exposés documenting financial improprieties and atrocious care of elderly residents. In addition, the Temporary State Commission on the Cost of Living conducted its own investigations on the nursing home industry in the state. In the foreword to the commission's final report (1975), the chairman of the commission, Andrew Stein, captured the tone of outrage about the abuses of this period:

> The dismal picture of venality and inhumanity painted by the proprietary nursing home industry shocked each and every member of the Commission. We found the proprietary nursing home system so riddled with corruption that it might not even be capable of complete reform. Accordingly, even as we strive to introduce desperately needed change, we must simultaneously enlarge and expand our non-profit system of care. It is necessary and proper, even taking into consideration guarantees that the proprietary system must end in this state. We cannot and must not continue to place the lives of our infirm elderly under the domination of a proprietary system that has so callously abused its trust. (Temporary State Commission 1975, 1–2)

State officials undertook a massive offensive. They stiffened fines, tightened regulations, conducted unannounced inspections, created graduated fines, produced public report cards, and tied reimbursement rates to the quality of care. More than 130 individuals were convicted of Medicaid fraud and related crimes. Most of the convictions involved fraudulent inclusions in their Medicaid cost reports. One operator, for example, billed more than $250,000 in personal expenditures to Medicaid. These expenditures included the purchase of a wedding cake, bridal gown, and flowers for his daughter and veterinary bills and shoeing expenses for his horses (Smith 1981, 101). Another operator included altered bills from an art dealer for Renoir, Utrillo, and Cassatt paintings used to decorate his mistress's apartment. In addition, forty-one individuals were convicted of kickback schemes involving nursing home operators and their suppliers (Smith 1981, 102). In 1976 proceedings were instituted to revoke the licenses of thirty-nine nursing home administrators (Smith 1981, 30).

Not surprisingly, New York was not subsequently viewed as a hospitable environment for nursing home innovation or for-profit development. State public health officials attempted to limit nursing home use by restricting expansion, providing expanded support for home care, and creating reimbursement incentives to encourage more restrictive use of nursing homes. More than a decade would pass before the aftershocks of the final disruptive events of the twentieth century would force even more radical change.

Aftershocks of the New Economy in the 1990s: The Reinvention of Care

In the 1990s, new shocks destabilized a system already shaken by earlier changes. Interrelated economic and political events now appear likely to trigger the final collapse of the nation's jerry-built system of long-term care. The introduction of Medicare and improvements in Social Security and private pensions produced a cumulative effect, reducing poverty rates among the elderly. In 1967 poverty rates among the over-sixty-five population was 30%, almost three times the poverty rate of eighteen-to-sixty-five-year-olds. However, by the mid-1990s the poverty rate of the elderly had dropped below 10%, slightly below that of eighteen-to-sixty-five-year-olds (De Lew 2000, 87). The elderly no longer appeared to be such a vulnerable population in need of protection. The ideology of the Internet and the global market revolution emerged in the 1990s, calling for greater competitiveness in order to survive in an increasingly global electronic marketplace. Welfare and entitlement programs, particularly for the elderly, were viewed as a threat to such competitiveness. The pervasiveness of this viewpoint produced, for the first time in the history of the United States, restriction in welfare and entitlement programs during a period of sustained economic growth. There were incentives to providers to shift care from indoor to outdoor forms of relief, which were assumed to be less costly. Following in the footsteps of New York's Medicaid program, many states adopted case-mix-adjusted or "resource utilization group" (RUG) reimbursement for nursing homes. Such payments provided nursing homes with a strong financial incentive to restrict utilization of their beds to heavy-care cases. In effect, RUG reimbursement shifted more routine care outside of the nursing home, just as "diagnostically related groups," a similar form of case-mix payment for hospitals in Medicare, had earlier shifted such care away from acute care hospitals. Similar changes in reimbursement were adopted for the Medicare program in the Balanced Budget Act of 1997. In the face of the combined effect of these payment incentives, nursing home population declined.

The Balanced Budget Act of 1997 also imposed an overall cap on Medicare payments to nursing homes, as well as payments for physical therapy and other services that had previously been paid on a fee-for-service basis—a loophole that had helped assure nursing home profitability. The financial impact of these changes devastated the industry, with five of the seven largest publicly traded nursing home chains beginning the new century operating under Chapter 11 bankruptcy protections (Dobson 2000).

The frail elderly and their families were also caught up in the aftershock of these changes. The personal and financial costs of long-term care continued to rise. Most individuals and their families faced the difficult choice of relying on their own informal family-based care, using out-of-pocket resources to pay for the accelerating catastrophic costs of the formal system of at-home or nursing home care, or accepting the stigma of indigence as a Medicaid recipient by spending down or transferring assets. However, a growing number of elderly and their families had the resources to pay for nursing home care but saw no reason to pay for something they did not want. The growing income and wealth inequalities of the elderly accelerated demands for an alternative to the demeaning accommodations of a welfare-driven system of care. The pressures of an aging population, a decline in the availability of informal caregivers, the erosion of public entitlements, and a decade of prosperity coalesced.

Entrepreneurs jumped on a large and growing opportunity. They reinvented care, and a new industry began to be defined. Privately financed assisted living developers tried to combine the elements of the old system into an attractive package that individuals and families would pay for. Assisted living was touted as the "killer application" of long-term care, and a development and investment boom began. This launched a new and troubling cycle of the old debate over how best to care for the frail elderly. The next chapter tells the story surrounding these developments.

3
Emergence of the Killer Application

The seeds for the killer application had been sown in the 1970s with the nursing home scandals and subsequent regulatory pressures. Some nursing home developers chose to switch from the traditional nursing home business to the seemingly greater freedom, simplicity, and profitability of private senior housing and boarding homes. They entered a diverse, fragmented market that was scattered even further on the periphery of the twentieth century's transformation of health institutions. Housing for seniors included homes for the elderly established by wealthy local philanthropists, fraternal lodges, and religious groups—remnants of the nineteenth century—as well as ma-and-pa private boarding homes developed in the late 1930s in the wake of the Social Security program that never made the transformation to nursing homes. These facilities were joined in the 1950s by the retirement communities of private developers in Florida and other locations that offered the promise of warmer winters and lower taxes. By the 1970s retirement developments like those in Florida had spread and began to dot the landscape on the suburban fringe of major urban centers. Low- and moderate-income elderly public and nonprofit housing developments, supported by Department of Housing and Urban Development financing and other public sources, began to add to this mix in the late 1960s. In the 1980s a curious mix of newcomers joined that diverse and disorganized market. They included freelancing real estate entrepreneurs from the early days of the publicly traded nursing homes in the 1970s. They were joined by individuals without any previous background in long-term care, including real estate developers of shopping malls and office buildings and those representing banks and investment interests. Perhaps most importantly, however, they were joined by missionary zealots motivated in part by their own personal experiences with the choices available to them in caring for an elderly relative. Convinced that they could provide better care at far less cost, they devoted their lives to doing just that.

Toward the end of the 1980s, those seeking to gain a foothold in the senior housing and adult care market were like wild animals drawn by the bright lights of the health care system. They crouched in the darkness united by two things: a desire for recognition and a fundamental antagonism toward the current health system providers. The time for attack was near.

Terry and Paul Klaassen seemed unlikely commanders to participate in such an attack. The story of their own operation bridges the generation between the older, familiar pattern of husband-and-wife teams that operated boarding homes for seniors and the brasher more aggressive newcomer developers. The decision to operate a facility, as it had been for many others, was in part motivated by their own experiences in getting assistance for elderly relatives in grim and impersonal nursing homes. It was also motivated by the relative attractiveness of the senior housing arrangements in Holland, which Paul had been exposed to when he visited his grandparents. A *verzorgingsehuzen*, or senior housing arrangement, provided for their care in a personalized homelike environment. The system of care for the frail elderly developed by New York's first settlers from Holland was about to return.

In 1981 the Klaassens sold their home and moved into a boarded-up nursing home in northern Virginia. They had a vision of creating a facility similar to the ones in Holland. They added two other nursing home conversions and then, in 1987, built their first prototype facility from scratch. It has a Victorian mansion style, capturing the flavor of that earlier era, but was designed with a different purpose in mind. It became the trademark for their company, Sunrise Assisted Living, Inc., and a prototype for the emerging assisted living industry.

An industry, or a movement, or whatever it was, however, needed a voice. Existing national trade organizations were at best ambivalent about these less-professional old-timers and renegade upstarts. The American Health Care Association, the national trade association of the for-profit nursing home industry, was not interested in diluting its advocacy by adding providers it regarded as heirs to the boarding home industry. The American Association for Homes for the Aged, while more sympathetic to the vision of assisted living, had a membership representing voluntary providers that had been historically hostile to for-profit operators. With a mixture of entrepreneurialism and missionary zeal that had driven the development of his company, Klaassen kept pushing. The National Association of Residential Care Facilities (NARCF) was the remaining trade association that had potential to become a kind of advocate and promoter of Klaassen's vision. Residential care facilities as the association defined them were "social models" of care, which provided housing, meals, and personal services in a family atmosphere and a setting similar to a private residence for the frail elderly, the developmentally disabled, and the mentally and physically impaired. It represented the fragmented inheritors of the deinstitutionalization or outdoor relief movement of the 1960s. It had many members who shared a similar vision, but the organization had a shoestring budget, no full-time staff, and no lobbying presence in Washington.

Having identified NARCF as the best target for a takeover, it seemed to Klaassen a simple matter of making them an offer they couldn't refuse. Carol Fisk, who was appointed by President Reagan as commissioner on aging, became enamored of the idea of assisted living. When she left office, she offered to work with Klaassen on his project. Klaassen offered to fund an office for NARCF, staffed by Fisk in Washington, for the first two years. He was invited to present his proposal at the annual national board meeting in Tulsa, Oklahoma, in September 1989. His proposal produced a heated controversy within the board, which resulted in the removal of his proposal from the agenda.

Klaassen, however, didn't walk away from the Tulsa meeting empty-handed. Three board members resigned on the spot in protest and walked out of the meeting, bumping into Klaassen, who had been waiting outside in the foyer. "I had struck out without even coming to the plate and so the four of us decided to make the best of it and go out to dinner," Klaassen would explain years later. "The doorman directed us to what he said was the best Lebanese restaurant in Tulsa. It was the only one" (Klaassen 2000). The Assisted Living Federation of America (ALFA) was formed with four members at the restaurant. Its initial headquarters were in the garage behind Klaassen's home, the same one that served as the original headquarters for Sunrise Assisted Living, Inc. Support was solicited from many of the individuals who were leaders in the new for-profit industry. Fisk was appointed the first director and Klaassen its first president. It soon eclipsed NARCF. A decade later it had 7,000 members, 37 state affiliates, and an annual budget of $5.8 million. Five years after the founding of ALFA, an industry that had lacked a name claimed revenues of almost $15 billion and between 30,000 and 40,000 facilities. Some analysts forecasted near exponential growth for the industry and projected that the assisted living industry revenues might exceed $30 billion by 2000 (Koss-Feder 1997, 36).

Assisted living had become the darling of Wall Street, and capital for expansion flowed freely. Headlines in the trade press trumpeted its virtues with such headlines as "Where There's Gray There's Green" and "Turning Silver into Gold." Assisted living companies indeed had a great story to sell. It had six key talking points: (1) The eighty-five-and-older population would grow by 43% in the 1990s and was projected to grow even faster in the years to follow. (2) The supply of nursing home beds per 1,000 of the eighty-five-and-older population would decline, as would the availability of informal care from adult children, who were increasingly geographically separated from their parents and members of double-wage-earner households in which neither spouse was free to provide care to parents. (3) The eighty-five-plus population that could afford private-market assisted living was growing at an even faster rate than the eighty-five-plus population as a whole. (4) Reimbursement pressures would continue to push more of those requiring less intensive care out of the hospitals and nursing homes. (5) Creating a lower-cost, more attractive alternative to private nursing home care was feasible because no one wanted to go to a nursing home, and regulatory and staffing requirements had pushed costs to a prohibitive level. (6) Investors, after facilities were filled, could expect a return of 30% to 50% on their investment. At the same time, traditional forms of real estate investment had become far less attractive. Office buildings were still suffering from the glut in supply created by the real estate boom in the 1980s that produced the savings and loan bankruptcies, and the strong investor interest in apartments had bid down the yield.

The blessing and the curse of assisted living was that its story was mostly true. As is typical with the boom-and-bust cycles of real estate and the stock market, the new industry was suddenly inundated with a tidal wave of capital for expansion. Individuals with some management experience and a good track record who could convince investors of both the enormous growth potential of the market and their ability to provide an extremely desirable product had access to a substantial flow of Wall Street money. Small regional family-based operations took advantage of these conditions by making initial public offerings of stock. Two companies, Sunrise Assisted Living and Kapson Senior Quarters, illustrate the chaotic ride that then ensued.

Sunrise Assisted Living, Inc., in its initial public offering in June 1996 announced plans to open fifty-five new assisted living communities by the end of 1999. That offering and a second offering later that year raised

$195 million to help the planned expansion. "Compassion Pays," read the headline of *Forbes* profile on the Klaassens and Sunrise operations ("Compassion Pays" 1997). Wall Street was convinced as well. A building and acquisitions frenzy ensued. There was a seemingly unending supply of capital flowing from venture capital firms, stock offerings, bank mortgages, joint ventures with local investors, and sale and long-term leasebacks and management contracts with other less experienced owners. Sunrise Assisted Living, Inc., a company that had begun in 1981 with financing from the sale of the Klaassens' home and the purchase of a boarded-up nursing home, encompassed an empire valued at $1.1 billion in 2000, operating 148 facilities in 23 states and the United Kingdom, with a total capacity for 5,621 elderly residents (Sunrise Assisted Living 2000).

Kapson Senior Quarters, however, had a more difficult ride. It had evolved out of a similar family-owned business passed on through three generations of Kaplans. Their story, however, developed into a complex and implausible soap opera involving a local family-operated adult home development company, one of the nation's largest publicly held nursing home conglomerates, and one of Wall Street's largest investment banks.

The Kaplans' family business began as a private adult home established on Long Island in the 1930s. With the additional income supplied by Social Security and the relative affluence of the area, the business prospered. Real estate holdings expanded under the management of the founder's son. In 1972 he began the development of what would become assisted living facilities. In 1985 those holdings were passed on to his three sons—Glenn, Wayne, and Evon—and the new business, Kapson Senior Quarters, focused exclusively on assisted living. By 1996 the Kaplans owned or managed 15 facilities with a capacity for 2,392 residents. Even though the Kaplans had achieved considerable success, they had bigger plans. Their initial public offering in June 1996, at the same time as Sunrise's initial public offering, brought in about $36 million to finance their expansion and to consolidate their ownership of the facilities that they currently managed. A subsequent preferred-stock offering of $50 million in July 1997 helped them further consolidate their ownership of facilities and begin construction or renovation of new properties.

Up to the time of those stock offerings, the Kaplans' story of growth and development mirrored that of the Klaassens and Sunrise, but then the story turns Byzantine. Enter Lazard Freres Real Estate Investors

(LFREI), the New York–based affiliate of the international investment bank Lazard Freres and Company, LLC, which manages over $2 billion in real estate investments. The stakes get higher and a ferocious struggle begins. Unlike stockholders, Lazard Freres's real estate principals become directly involved in managing and growing a business. They assumed that they would be able to sell the business in five to seven years at a substantial profit, either through sale to another national assisted living company or through a new public offering of stock. Their plan was to create a dominant national player in the rapidly growing assisted living sector. To Lazard Freres, Kapson Senior Quarters, heavily leveraged and operating at a loss as a result of its expansion efforts, was tantalizing prey.

In the resulting complex financial and legal interrelationships used to implement its strategy, Lazard Freres spun out of control. In July 1997, through its affiliate Prometheus Assisted Living, LLC, LFREI announced plans to invest an additional $135 million in ARV Assisted Living, Inc., of Costa Mesa, California, which would give a LFREI a 49.9% stake as a shareholder in ARV. ARV, a firm founded in 1980, operated forty-nine facilities with a total of 6,300 units concentrated in California, Florida, and the Midwest. At the same time, LFREI was in the process of buying out Kapson Senior Quarters for about $250 million, including the assumption of its debts. The initial plan was that LFREI would take a controlling position on the board of Kapson, the management would remain unchanged, and a strategic alliance would be formed with ARV. "Our investment in Kaplan dramatically expands our presence in the assisted living industry and demonstrates our commitment to one of the fastest growing segments of the health industry," said Arthur P. Solomon, chairman and senior managing director of LFREI. "Assuming the alliance with ARV is established, the two companies will become the largest owners and operators of assisted living facilities in the country" (PR Newswire 1997, 2). Lazard Freres amended its offer, reducing the purchase price by $20 million to $230 million, and tendering an offer to purchase all of the Kapson stock shares for $180 million and to assume approximately $50 million of the company's debt.

Kapson Senior Quarters, now privately owned by LFREI, caught sight of new prey. Atria Communities, Inc., had originally been a wholly owned subsidiary of Vencor, the largest publicly traded nursing home chain in the nation, based in Lexington, Kentucky. It had been spun off from Vencor in 1996, but Vencor still owned 43% of its stock and needed cash.

Vencor's own acquisition binge had included a $1.4 billion stock swap for the acquisition of the Hill Haven nursing home chain in 1995 and the $638 million acquisition of Transitional Hospitals Corporation in 1997. However, in 1998 Vencor hit a wall. Its net reported loss from operations in 1998 was $573 million, which violated the financial covenants of its $1 billion dollar bank credit. The impact of the 1997 Balanced Budget Act on Medicare ancillary revenues and the demands by the Health Care Financing Administration for repayment of $1.3 billion in what it claimed were fraudulent overpayments since 1992 cast a darkening shadow on the company. In September 1999, the inevitable could be avoided no longer, and Vencor filed for Chapter 11 bankruptcy protection. A company that had generated more than $3 billion in revenues in 1997 and operated 295 nursing homes with 38,753 licensed beds and 56 hospitals with 4,953 licensed beds was now a pauper. According to a July 30, 1999, Associated Press wire story, "Site of Vencor Will Go on Auction Block," the site for its planned corporate headquarters along with the architectural plans for an I. M. Pei–designed $60 million swirling twenty-five-story tower on the downtown riverfront in Louisville were put on the auction block in August 1999.

LFREI proceeded to cut a deal to purchase Atria Communities for $750 million and merge its operations with those of Kapson Senior Quarters. As a result, Vencor received approximately $177.5 million of badly needed cash. The deal, however, hit its first snag with a suit against LFREI by ARV for breach of contract, claiming right of first refusal in the acquisition. ARV claimed that the Atria deal could not proceed without the approval of 75% of the ARV board. LFREI was ARV's major stockholder, owning 47.9% of its stock. The plan for ARV to lease and operate the Kapson properties fell through because of a failure to reach agreement on the leasing rates. The lawsuit was subsequently decided in Lazard Freres's favor. That impediment out of the way, LFREI then proceeded to consolidate management and the back office operations of the merged firm in Lexington. C. Patrick Mulloy II, the new CEO of the merged firm, then proceeded to fire the Kaplan team "for cause." In response, the Kaplan team sued Lazard Freres, Atria, Mulloy, and others involved in the transaction for federal securities fraud and state claims for fraud, fraudulent inducement, and negligent misrepresentation. The suit was based on what they perceived to be the assurances offered by

Lazard Freres at the time of the purchase that they would manage the new company and receive shares in the newly formed company as part of their compensation. The suit was dismissed in district court on February 3, 2000. Adding to the turbulence, Lazard Freres was embroiled in its own internal power struggle between Arthur Solomon, the partner who ran LFREI, and the top brass at Lazard Freres. The struggle culminated in Solomon's departure. Another member of the real estate team was terminated, and a third resigned. Solomon sued Lazard Freres for breach of fiduciary duty and defamation of character. The suit was settled in June 1999 for terms that were not disclosed (Fulman 1999).

After the forced departure of Arthur Solomon, institutional investors who were limited partners in LFREI hired their own lawyer to explore options for limiting their commitment of funds. Those concerned about the management turnover included the director of investments for the $12 billion Howard Hughes Research Institute and the $101 billion California Teachers Retirement System.

As of June 2001, LFREI continues to struggle with a strategy that will allow it to recoup its assisted living investments in what is now a very deflated market. As one industry observer I interviewed noted in reviewing the wreckage of LFREI's vision of national assisted living real estate dominance, "I guess that's what you get in this industry when you combine twenty-something MBAs from a Wall Street investment bank, New York Jews, good old boys from Kentucky, and California surfers!"

These distant high-finance and top management intrigues permeated the day-to-day operations of facilities in sometimes unpredictable ways. Local administrators who remained after the transfer of ownership found the Louisville firm's effort to impose its own distinctive " signature" on Kapson's New York City facilities amusing. Part of the Kapson-managed facilities' "signature" was to have waiters and waitresses dressed in black ties and white shirts, just as residents might expect in upscale restaurants in the city. Atria's approach was to dress waitresses in flowered country smocks that had a "down home southern pancake cottage look." Both the staff and residents were offended by the changes, and in several cases it may have contributed to the termination of the management contracts with facilities owned by local investors.

All parties (Lazard Freres, Atria/Senior Quarters, Sunrise, Altera, and other publicly traded national firms), however, saw New York City as a ripe target for expansion. The region had lagged behind in assisted living development. It was as if a vacuum were waiting to be filled. The previous perception of a more hostile business climate for long-term care development, an aftermath of the nursing home scandals in the 1970s, had dampened development. With a Republican governor and mayor, the business climate had changed. Trade leaders estimated that about 20,000 private assisted living units would come on the market in the metropolitan area by the end of 2000 (Koss-Feder 1997, 36). Concerned about economic development, officials had begun to encourage assisted living development projects and to cut through red tape that had discouraged real estate development efforts in the past. Symbolic of the profound shift taking place was the Manhattan-based real estate firm Savanna Partners' proposed $75 million plan to renovate a landmark property to become "The Towers of Central Park West," a luxury assisted living complex. The property, originally opened as a cancer hospital in the 1880s by John Jacob Aster, previously housed Bernard Bergman's Towers Nursing Home in the 1950s and 1960s. State regulators forced its closure in 1974. As described in the previous chapter, financial improprieties and its failure to comply with state and federal nursing home standards brought notoriety to the facility and touched off a wave of nursing home investigations in New York State. It was now part of a new wave of speculative growth.

What Is Assisted Living?

In spite of a dramatic increase in private development and a massive influx of venture capital that flowed into assisted living, there is no local or national consensus on what it is. People cannot agree on what services are essential, who are appropriate recipients for such care, or what role state and local government should have, if any, in regulating such diverse private-market and publicly funded organizations. It is the proverbial blind men and the elephant problem, with the spokespersons for every provider group putting their own spin on developments. For example, home care agencies emphasize the program aspects of assisted living. That is, home care agencies define assisted living as a package of services not tied to any particular facility and argue that a variety of settings (e.g., private homes, boarding homes, retirement communities, etc.) can serve as appropriate facilities for such care. Facility provider associations, on the other hand, emphasize the importance of flexibility in responding to the individual needs of residents within facilities specifically designed to integrate housing and service delivery.

I argue, however, that the basic impediment to a clear definition of assisted living is that it simply does not fit into the existing organized arrangements for health care and services for the elderly. From a historical perspective, assisted living services and facilities are the culmination of events that have reshaped the organization and financing of care (Kane and Brown 1993). In the language of the information revolution, assisted living is a "killer application." Rather than fitting into the existing arrangements of care, it radically alters those arrangements. It alters them as radically as the microcomputer and the Internet have reshaped the organization of most businesses. Assisted living is an eclectic combination of medical, housing, hotel, and recreational services, promising the same increased value as software applications combining the functions of a variety of essential stand-alone applications.

A New Model for Organizing Care

The traditional medical and assisted living organizational models envision the flow of services to people and of funds to service providers in fundamentally different ways. The medical model envisions processing patients through a system with separate units or facilities providing specialized services to homogenous populations. That is the classical production model of scientific management that began to be embraced in the social and scientific transformation of medicine almost a century ago. It assumes that illnesses can be addressed through specialization of both practitioners and the settings in which care is provided. As the population has aged, medical needs have shifted from acute care interventions toward long-term management of multiple chronic conditions. Little, however, has changed in the organization of services to accommodate that shift. While much lip service is given to providing a "seamless continuum of care," the reality is a fragmented hodgepodge of services that are at best only loosely connected, overlapping, and in competition with each other and at the same time leave large gaps in service, as any adult who tries to patch something together to take care of his or her parents discovers. Care is organized for the convenience of those who have power, and the adult child who is organizing care for an elderly parent usually has little.

Some have attempted to address the obvious fragmentation of traditional ways of organizing care but with limited success. Continuing care retirement communities (CCRCs), an idea initially developed by the Society of Friends in Philadelphia in the 1960s, expanded nationally in the 1970s and 1980s. While embracing the traditional view of a continuum of specialized care (e.g., housing for independent living, personal care, and skilled nursing home units), CCRCs offer each type of service on a single campus. For an initial entrance fee and flat monthly charges, CCRCs offer a comprehensive care package to meet all of the residents' needs for the remainder of their lives. In spite of all the enthusiasm of experts, however, about fifty CCRCs either went bankrupt or faced financial difficulties that left their residents stranded without the care they had been promised and paid for (PR Newswire 1987). As a result, most states now have laws regulating CCRCs, which include a requirement that adequate reserves be maintained. Growth was slowed by the new regulations and by the resistance of prospective residents to the high entrance fees (Knox 1997). Nevertheless, there are currently more than two thousand CCRCs nationally.

At the low-income end, much effort has gone into attempting to integrate care by designing financial packages that combine Medicare and Medicaid payments; these efforts have culminated in the Programs of All-Inclusive Care for the Elderly (PACE), a national movement with programs in local communities. These programs, modeled after the San Francisco On Lok program, provide most of the care at day care sites for a flat combined Medicare and Medicaid rate. They have so far attracted almost no non-Medicaid-eligible subscribers, and they are likely to remain a small boutique program. Even the well-established and revered On Lok program in San Francisco has only 8% non-Medicaid private-pay enrollees (Bodenheimer 1999). A spokesperson for PACE stated that they have such a hard time recruiting even Medicaid-eligible subscribers that the luxury of "cream skimming," selectively admitting less costly applicants, doesn't exist for them (Bodenheimer 1999).

Thus, while PACE and the CCRCs offer an alternative to the traditional approaches to providing and paying for the care for the elderly, they do not alter power relationships between providers and recipients of care in the same way that assisted living claims to do. The facility, whether a nursing home or day care center, is the "home" of the provider of specialized services, and the patient or resident is the transient client, patient, or guest.

Yet patients and their families have made many inroads that have cracked the calcified provider-dominated structure of care. Their efforts to effect change are testimony both to their resilience in insisting on control over their own lives and the power of the market in forcing accommodation to such demands. Two such changes, the creation of birthing centers and hospice programs, illustrate the same complex dynamics now influencing the emergence and evolution of assisted living.

Birthing centers grew out of the childbirth education movement. The movement traces its roots to the efforts of New York City's Maternity Center Association in the 1940s. The association developed childbirth education classes and promoted natural childbirth (Burst 1987). Nineteen forty marked the end of the transition from the nineteenth-century pattern, in which births took place in the home with female family members or midwives in attendance, to the twentieth-century practice of a seemingly scientific, sterile assembly line environment that passed the woman through an admissions office, waiting room, active labor room, delivery room, recovery room, and hospital room. In this environment, women give birth in the company of strangers, heavily sedated and unconscious, and managed by aloof male obstetricians. Concern about the safety of the mother and infant motivated this shift in the location of care. Objective assessments at the time suggested that whatever improvements in safety were gained by the change in location were offset by the increases in the use of anesthesia, forceps, and other instruments, which were encouraged by the ease of their availability in hospitals (Leavitt 1983, 299). The women's movement in the 1960s and 1970s added fuel to that concern. One response was the growth of nurse midwifery. The major changes in hospital-provided services, however, came in the 1980s, when declining hospital occupancy and competition for market share heated up. Almost every hospital with a large obstetrical service developed "family-centered" obstetrical care options. As an early innovator, Rush-Presbyterian Hospital in Chicago, for example, developed a birth center in 1979. It provided mothers with low-risk pregnancies the opportunity to have their babies in a simulated homelike environment, but adjacent to the hospital's delivery neonatal care areas. Labor, delivery, and immediate neonatal care all took place in a birth center "apartment." A study that compared the outcomes of birth center care to the outcomes of conventional care births found no difference in the outcomes (Waskerwitz et al. 1985). As the risks have become better understood, hospital-based birthing centers have faced increasing competition from freestanding ones, which are operated by more entrepreneurial obstetricians and midwifery teams. One such operation in California, developed by a board-certified obstetrician and gynecologist, offers suites with double beds and two private baths. Also, the expectant parents can share a sunny tiled patio courtyard with a fountain and a country kitchen abundantly stocked with healthy snacks (Harper 2001). State licensing and health insurance payment restrictions are the only forces slowing the increase in freestanding birthing centers that compete with traditional hospital obstetrical services.

A precursor to the assisted living movement, the hospice movement emerged in the 1960s as a reaction to the depersonalized care received by the dying in hospitals. Most hospitals failed to address adequately the pain and discomfort associated with cancer and its treatment. Early advocates of the hospice movement urged more humanistic and holistic treatment that included greater attention to palliative care and to the psychosocial needs of patients and their families. They sought constructive alternatives when more aggressive treatment offered no hope. The early efforts were community-based nonprofit organizations that relied on a network of volunteers. From their beginnings as a loosely connected reform movement, hospices have evolved into well-defined organizations that are well integrated into the traditional care system. While the first hospices were freestanding operations, most have now become either home health agency-based or hospital-based programs. They began to attract support from the National Cancer Institute and private philanthropies in the 1970s. In 1977 they formed their own association, the National Hospice Organization (NHO), to promote education, common standards, and, of course, third-party payment. NHO realized the latter objective with the passage of federal legislation in 1982 that made hospices eligible to receive payment under the Medicare program and the subsequent amendment in 1985 to this law that made them eligible to receive Medicaid payments. The for-profit home health chains, predictably, entered the hospice market shortly afterwards. What had begun as an idealistic volunteer movement completed its transformation into a business and into a fully integrated component of the existing care system (Paradis and Cummings 1986). The number of clients cared for by hospice programs grows at a rate of 13% a year, a growth rate unrivaled by any other segment of health care (Gillen 1995, 28). Yet in the process of growing, hospices ceased to be synonymous with the broader holistic vision of palliative care.

Market forces in the health care sector, with or without a social movement, can move institutions away from assembly-line, provider-centered care to care provided in a single setting more controlled by the patient. For example, some hospital emergency departments, faced with increasing competition from stand-alone urgent care centers and other hospitals, have redesigned their services to achieve a simplified patient flow. In most of these redesigned emergency services, a single private room serves as a waiting, triage, diagnosis, and treatment room. Patients and their families like these changes. It gives them a greater sense of privacy and a feeling of more personalized care. They feel less like they are being processed on a conveyor belt. It reduces the stress produced by a sense of loss of control. They are in charge.

Nowhere is the argument for organizing care around the patient more inherently logical than in the area of long-term care. One could argue that forced transfers of the frail elderly can kill them. The results of studies support the "transfer trauma" hypothesis, i.e., that death rates rise in the first few months after a patient is transferred to a nursing home (Thorson 1988). One study noted an increase in fall rates of nursing home residents after relocation to a new facility (Freidman et al. 1995). Other studies have noted that patients suffering from dementia are more seriously affected by relocation (Bredin et al. 1995; Roberston et al. 1995). Adequate preparation and postdischarge orientation programs as well as the degree to which the resident can exercise control and choice in such relocations appear to mitigate some of the adverse outcomes (Cohen 1986). The risk of transfer trauma has even been used, although unsuccessfully, as an argument in legal efforts to block the closure of substandard nursing homes by state regulators (*O'Bannon v. Town Court Nursing Center* 1980).

None of what I have described here with regard to ways of reorganizing care reflects new insights into what patients want or what is in their best interests. For the most part, the organization of care usually reflects the relative power of the participants. Change in organization is the result of change in power. Powerful patients, a Rose Kennedy or a Ronald Reagan, are not processed through a "continuum of care." Their care, whatever that entails, is at their family's beck and call and in their own home. The only exception is highly specialized care, such as surgery to correct a broken hip, which temporarily reduces the power of even so powerful a client. Until the 1930s, most physicians treated their private patients in the patient's home. The twentieth-century transformation of medicine produced a shift in power and, partly as a consequence, a shift in the location of care.

The shift in the location and organization of care in the assisted living model, however, symbolizes a far more profound conflict with the traditional medical model. It challenges the basis upon which choices about care are made. Services in the private-market assisted living model flow to the recipient based not on the assessments of needs by health professionals but on the desires and preferences of the residents or their family. The private-market assisted living model places emphasis on the right of recipients to assume risk for the choices they make, a necessary precondition for "aging in place," a value touted as a key benefit of assisted living. In contrast, the medical model, with all its more recent efforts to accommodate the wishes of the patient and family, emphasizes the delegation of such decisions to professionals responsible for reducing medical risks to their lowest possible level. In short, the assisted living decision-making model bypasses all of the elaborate public and professional controls regarding what standards are required of those who provide services, what those services entail, who is eligible to receive them, and how they are to be paid for. The strength of the private-market assisted living model is its flexibility in designing and packaging services best able to attract what it defines as its "customers."

As the brief history of care in the previous chapter explains, long-term care evolved into a very different institutional culture than hospitals. Even after they were no longer simply almshouses, nursing homes served as the handmaidens of the acute care sector. It was a place to send the "GOMERS" (the "Get out of my emergency room" patients) who did not lend themselves to interesting or profitable treatment. Like the back wards of a psychiatric hospital, nursing homes and other long-term care arrangements served as a dumping ground. More recently, acute care providers have viewed them as supply reservoirs to help keep their own acute care beds filled. Some hospitals began to acquire nursing homes in the 1990s. Some developed more elaborate feeder systems that also included personal care facilities and senior housing. The feeder systems were justified not as a way to allow people to age in place but as a way to protect market share by generating acute care admissions.

The private assisted living movement tends to reverse the power in the relationship between the provider and the person needing care. This is described as "customer empowerment," that is, creating an environment that rewards individuals for figuring out what customers are willing to pay for and giving them what they want. While care coordination, for example, may be provided as a part of the package of services offered to residents, the ultimate decision in terms of what services are purchased is made by the resident or responsible family members. Most people do not want to be uprooted from familiar surroundings, family, and friends or to surrender control of their lives to others. Most, of course, prefer their own communities to an artificial one. Most will uproot themselves only when growing infirmities force such relocations. A basic marketing strategy of assisted living facilities is to provide, as much as possible, the look and feel of attractive private housing and thus to ease the frail elderly person's resistance to relocation.

Why the Traditional Health Care Providers Can't Compete

If this is all so obvious, why haven't hospitals and nursing homes changed more to address these needs? The answer is that hospitals and nursing homes are, to a large extent, the captives of the third parties that pay their bills. Form follows the money. Insurance payments shape how hospitals and nursing homes organize care. Commercial insurance companies, Blue Cross plans, Medicare, and Medicaid account for most of their income. Thus, those providers must march to the drum of insurance carriers. From the perspective of an insurance company, an insurable risk is an event that is rare, costly, undesired, and unpredictable. An insurance company worries about "moral hazard," that is, the ability of an insured person (or welfare beneficiary) to anticipate medical needs and use insurance to his or her advantage. As a result, insurance companies were at first reluctant to write policies to cover health care costs, because many of the expenses are predictable, not catastrophic in nature, and even desirable to the insured. For example, patients might like and encourage their physician to prescribe a couple of extra hospital days to rest and recuperate after major surgery or the birth of a child.

Insurance carriers also control their costs by limiting coverage to precisely defined medical conditions and to services provided only by appropriately licensed and credentialed providers. Nursing homes, as I noted earlier, became increasingly medicalized facilities after the passage of Medicare and Medicaid, as services followed the path, laid out by the insurance companies, leading to the dollars.

In addition, although insurers will not come right out and say it, they prefer to cover services and procedures that are unpleasant. For example, health insurance plans are more likely to cover electroconvulsive shock than psychotherapy, back surgery than massage, and skilled nursing home care than personal care assistance in one's home. It is not because insurers are sadistic or even that they wish to limit payments to services that have demonstrated their effectiveness. They are simply trying to run a business and control their expenses. Who would not like to have a kind, patient listener to talk with about his problems, an attentive massage for her sore back, and an aide to do the dishes and make meals for free? The insured and their providers have always been resourceful in using the insurance system to get what they want. How can an insurance company determine who can or cannot be permitted to receive such services and from whom? Such proposed benefits give insurance executives and actuaries nightmares.

Thus, the financing of long-term care through health insurance encourages the creation of medicalized homogeneous organizations for care that essentially perpetuate the almshouse stigma. A move toward making nursing homes more attractive and less stigmatized would increase their desirability and the costs borne by insurance. It is hard to serve two masters. Most assisted living developers are scornful of the timid and incomplete efforts of traditional health care providers to compete in the assisted living market. They recount the florescent lights, sterile corridors, and intimidating medical atmosphere in some of the attempts to convert facilities for the private assisted living market. "It's a real marketing challenge! People need to have a reason to get out of bed," said one assisted living executive I interviewed.

In contrast, private assisted living developers focus on those who pay for goods and services out of their own pockets. They embrace the housing and hospitality model rather than the medical and insurance model of care. Their job is to figure out what individual customers, not insurance companies, will pay for and to provide it. There is a liberating feeling to this approach that most health care providers envy. The credentials and the licensing of providers are less important. Private assisted living eliminates all the third parties and middlemen: the insurance companies, the professional licensing boards and credentialing bodies, the state facility licensing agencies, and most of the inspectors. What is left is a contract between the assisted living organization and the resident. The key is to provide the customer with something that he or she needs and that looks like a good value. It is a simpler business. If you fill enough units and if you can keep your cost down, you make a profit. You don't need to worry about caring for people who cannot afford to pay you or about collecting payments from third parties. If a person is disruptive or too difficult to care for in your community, you don't need to care for him or her. When you add to this the combination of low interest rates and rising real estate values, you have an attractive business to be in. It is one free of the constraints of insurance controls.

The Killer Application Advantage

Health-related providers in the 1990s faced elaborate requirements that slowed or restricted expansion through certificate-of-need limits, third-party contract restrictions, and other forms of regulatory and contractual oversight. The sources of capital that health care providers have depended upon to expand or replace facilities (earnings from operations, capital payments from third parties, endowments, bonds, and commercial loans) have shrunk. Capital payments have been increasingly restricted, and earnings from operations have plummeted. Most state Medicaid programs have restricted or reduced nursing home capital cost payments and some, such as Pennsylvania, have even ceased to reimburse new nursing homes for capital costs. Most new integrated delivery systems have invested heavily in the acquisition of physician practices and other facilities. This has hampered their ability to incur further indebtedness. The 1998 $1.3 billion bankruptcy of the Allegheny Health System in Philadelphia, which included eight hospitals and employed more than seventeen thousand people, provided another object lesson in the risks of aggressive acquisition strategies (Burns et al. 2000).

In contrast, assisted living developers in the 1990s had much easier access to capital, as the stories of Sunrise Assisted Living and Kapson Senior Quarters illustrated. Low interest rates and rising prices in the housing market made real estate an increasingly attractive investment. In the 1990s real estate investment trusts (REITs), for example, provided an expanding attractive source of funds. REITs were originally created in the 1960s as a way for moderate-income investors to participate in the real estate market. Rather than investing directly in real estate, the investor purchases shares in an REIT. In return the investors receive dividends equivalent to 95% of the taxable rental income generated from properties owned by the trust. The value of the shares rises as the value of the real estate properties rises and as real estate prices in general rise.

In the mid-1990s there was more than $150 billion invested in REITs, and at that time the amount was doubling every one and a half years. The advantage such arrangements provided for assisted living developers was an almost unlimited source of capital for rapid expansion without assuming additional debt. Such "black box" or "off-balance-sheet" financing became an increasingly attractive option for publicly traded long-term care and assisted living companies (Japsen 1998, 76). These were arrangements similar to those made notorious by the Enron bankruptcy in 2001. The advantages of such off-balance-sheet financing disappear when growth slows. While REITs increase access to capital, they also increase the financial risk with a level of indebtedness that is much greater than is apparent from the balance sheet. Separating ownership of the real estate from ownership of the assisted living operation works fine as long as the investment is profitable for all parties. Costly legal wrangling results, however, if adverse conditions force the investment to be unwound. In financial terms, the costs of financial distress are substantially increased when asset repackaging becomes necessary. Those costs may offset the gains from easier access to capital. Publicly traded assisted living firms can also acquire capital through stock offerings, and such equity investments provide some buffer against market shocks. Yet many health professionals express concern about the conflict equity investment may pose between meeting the needs of investors and meeting the needs of assisted living residents.

However, the private-market assisted living facilities do not merely compete with traditionally organized care services; they feed off of them. This is the institutional version of the "cream skimming" scenario described in Chapter 1 that exists between New York and Florida. Private-market assisted living attracts people with higher incomes who can afford the private-market rates and require less care away from hospitals and nursing homes. When they run out of money or become too costly to care for, they can be discharged to nursing homes and hospitals. As a result, hospitals and nursing homes face caring for an increasing share of indigent patients who are more costly to care for. The private assisted living facilities absorb the profits, and the more traditional providers of health care absorb the increasing losses. A death spiral could begin, with the parasites eventually killing the hosts. In addition, assisted living facilities can, through their role in providing care coordination for their residents, further enhance their bargaining advantage by negotiating contracts on their residents' behalf for services from health care providers.

The Battle for Control of the Market

Table 3.1 summarizes the advantages and disadvantages of the traditional medical/insurance and private-market assisted living models. The advantage of the traditional medical/insurance model is that it ensures well-established standards of care, established methods of regulation, and at least some limited commitment to equal basic treatment regardless of income. In contrast, the private assisted living model lacks any agreed-upon measurable standards, has limited regulation, and ignores issues related to equity in access. The disadvantages often attributed to the traditional medical model are that it tends to be unresponsive to those being served, to be more costly, and to suffer increasingly from a lack of quick access to capital to respond to market demands. In contrast,

Table 3.1 Medical/Insurance vs. Assisted Living Models

	Medical/Insurance Model	Assisted Living Model
Market responsiveness	Unresponsive: fragmented, rigid, costly, and insurance dependent	Responsive: flexible, customer driven, and "empowering"
Regulatory oversight of services	Well-defined services with clear, accepted standards of care and methods of monitoring that care	Lack of standards, potential for abuse
Regulatory oversight of financing	Extensive: heavily regulated rates and control of expansion	Little: inherently unstable boom and bust cycles
Access to capital	Slow and increasingly limited	Quick and, in boom times, almost unlimited capital
Commitment to a single standard of care	Commitment to a single minimal standard of care and at least partial mainstreaming of care to low-income groups	None: private development focused primarily on higher-income groups

the private-market assisted living model seems better tailored to meet the wishes of its customers and has had better access to the capital markets.

The Eye of the Storm

Thus the emergence of assisted living, the killer application, is both exhilarating and terrifying. It is at the intersection of the conflicting forces shaping health and housing policies in the United States. It is in the eye of the looming storm.

Public health officials, health care professionals, and hospital and nursing home operators may be quick to dismiss the private assisted living movement as an old quack nostrum repackaged in a new bottle on a larger scale. Public health officials have fought battles against patent medicines and quack healers for a long time. They have closed down many sanitariums operated by cultists and unscrupulous operators preying on the public by promising results that are impossible to deliver.

Yet the more one investigates, the harder it is to separate the good actors from the bad ones. We face more complex problems that deal with basic questions about social class, the nature of communities, and ultimately, the kind of society we fear we will become. Embedded in all the activity surrounding assisted living development are some of the better answers.

In the previous chapter I traced the social history of care for the frail elderly. Three seemingly irresolvable tensions over its purpose, organization, and importance persist. The new killer application has emerged to challenge the dominance of the traditional medical/insurance model. There is both a pessimistic and an optimistic scenario for how this struggle will be resolved.

The pessimistic scenario is that the growing ascendancy of the private assisted living model will return the organization of care for the elderly to that which existed in the nineteenth century. It will force the demise of the traditional providers of acute and long-term care. During the nineteenth century, middle- and upper-income persons were cared for in their own homes. Public and voluntary hospitals (that is, public almshouses and their private charitable equivalents) exclusively provided care for the poor. It is likely that, as a cost-saving measure for the depleted traditional medical care system, much of the care for the frail elderly poor will be shifted to something called "assisted living." However, without the standards that have been put in place in health-related institutions or the market power that private assisted living customers are potentially able to exert on service providers, many may be subjected to scandalous conditions. The abuses that have plagued the indigent boarding home industry as well as its predecessors in the eighteenth- and nineteenth-century almshouses may return to haunt us on a larger scale.

The optimistic scenario is that a synthesis will be achieved between the two models that will assure minimum levels of care and that will take advantage of the strengths of both. Such a synthesis will not be easy to achieve. The history of caring for the frail elderly in the United States is replete with examples of unanticipated consequences of the best-intentioned changes in the health and social service system having disastrous effects. The basic questions faced now by health services researchers, regulators, traditional service providers, and financial institutions, to say nothing of the frail elderly themselves and their families, essentially take us back to all the issues faced in the history of licensure, regulation, and financing of health-related services in the United States.

Does it really work the way I have suggested, or have I just created straw men? Can we take at face value what health professionals and industry developers say about assisted living? In the next section I will describe with concrete examples the day-to-day efforts of the frail elderly to control their lives in such settings and the struggles of assisted living operators to expand their share of the long-term care market.

Part II
The Struggle for Control over Markets and Lives

4
Markets, Margin, and Mission

The great American dream of serving humanity while making large profits flourished as a driving force behind the development of assisted living in the 1990s. Yet even missionaries unconcerned about profits need a margin of income greater than expenses. "No margin, no mission," as they say in the nonprofit sector. This chapter describes how developers try to achieve both. It looks inside the killer application described in the previous chapter.

Conceiving of assisted living either as a profitable large business or a missionary social reform movement required a fertile imagination prior to the 1990s. The boarding home sector seemed to have little earning potential and a bad reputation. Boarding homes made headlines when fires killed elderly residents. The operators often made a marginal living. Some were widows who rented out rooms. One provider in New Jersey was a poultry farmer whose chickens stopped laying eggs when a drag strip was built next door. He converted the chicken coop to rooms for discharged psychiatric patients and elderly persons covered by Supplemental Security Income (SSI). Some were kindhearted and well meaning, others callous and crooked. At best, residential care for the frail elderly was a small-time mom-and-pop business. Envisioning a service industry that would combine the characteristics of the hotel and fast-food chain franchises of the 1950s, the hospital and nursing home chains of the 1960s and the upper-income retirement developments of the 1970s took imagination. Envisioning that service industry as part of a social movement bent on radically altering the existing health system took an even more fertile imagination.

In this chapter I describe how assisted living works as a business. It is divided into two sections. The first provides an overview of the basic strategy of the business. The second section examines the mission of assisted living.

Markets and Margin

Assisted living is a competitive business. Competition produces winners and losers. The winners in the assisted living business pick the right locations; get adequate, affordable financing; and effectively manage the myriad of day-to-day details involved in operations. These achievements are easy things to say, but harder to accomplish, particularly in an urban environment.

Picking the Right Locations

Location, location, location, as the cliché goes, are the keys to success in sales. Developers do market feasibility studies to pick the right sites. They look for areas with a growing, affluent population. Many will target areas not with affluent elderly households but with a concentration of affluent forty-five-to-sixty-five-year-olds. They are looking for successful two-career professional families likely to assume responsibility for an aging parent soon. National developers start by scanning demographics for likely regional targets. Some local developers, more familiar with an area, will scan real estate ads and prowl promising neighborhoods and then put together demographic statistics almost as an afterthought to give a degree of comfort to skeptical and often remote potential financial backers.

If the numbers or the developers' instincts suggest promise, then the developers, or the consulting firms they hire to assist them, look at potential competitors. They look at existing nursing homes and adult homes as well as other assisted living facilities. They may talk to hospital discharge planers and home health agencies about their referral patterns and placement problems. Newly opened facilities absorb more local demand as they fill up. This will affect other facilities that enter the market, since they face deficit financing until most of their units are rented. They either meet projections during the "fill-up" stage or face absorbing unanticipated deficits. Mistakes will jeopardize financing of future projects; too many mistakes will force a developer into bankruptcy. The nature of the business is such that filled facilities don't compete head-to-head on a day-to-day basis. The average length of stay of residents may be three years or more, so a one-hundred unit facility will generate on the average only two or three openings a month. Unlike families with elderly relatives on waiting lists for retirement communities, families looking for an assisted living placement typically cannot wait. The operator of a facility filled to capacity is often willing to refer prospective clients to other facilities on the assumption that the favor will be returned in the future.

A developer will try to do a thorough job of sizing up competitors. Often they or those that they have hired to do the market feasibility study will schedule visits to the facilities in the service area and talk with managers. They check out the pricing arrangements, admission and discharge criteria, and amenities and services offered by the facility. Many operators assume that they might as well be up front about sharing such information. If they do not, their competitors will employ "mystery shoppers," elderly relatives or friends whom developers or their consultants hire to gather information by posing as potential customers. This provides some senior citizens with an amusing diversion and others with adventurous new careers as "spies," a role at which some become very adept.

The goal of this process is to determine how a new facility will fit into a community, given its pricing, amenities, and market niche. Developers are willing to pay a premium for visible, accessible sites and prestige addresses with attractive grounds and commanding views. Such locations are in marked contrast to the locations of traditional nursing and boarding homes.

The ratio of the number of licensed long-term care beds to the number of elderly in an area is used as an indicator of supply in feasibility studies. Adult homes, skilled nursing facilities, and hospitals siphon off a segment of an assisted living facility's market. Nursing homes or hospitals with excess capacity may consider conversions or develop respite and home care programs, thus absorbing some of the middle ground in the long-term care market that could be occupied by assisted living facilities.

In New York City, for example, except for Staten Island (the least densely populated borough in the city) and the Bronx (which has historically provided many of the nursing home beds for the city's low-income population), these statistics indicate that there is considerable room for expansion of assisted living care. The projected growth in the over-eighty-five population in the remaining boroughs also makes these areas look attractive for development. At best, however, the potential private assisted living market is only the top third of the income distribution, elderly households with incomes greater than $25,000 a year. Given New York City prices, perhaps only the 5% of those over the age of eighty-five, those with household incomes over $100,000, are really qualified prospects. Only Manhattan, home to almost half of New York City's households with incomes over $100,000, meets this requirement. There are also many unlicensed private retirement housing complexes in the city, which do not show up in the licensed bed statistics. Further, there were more than thirteen new assisted living projects in 2000, with more than twelve hundred units still under construction (Jackson and Acks 2000). These statistics also fail to take into account the distinctive dynamics of the housing market in New York City. Rent control and co-op housing effectively provide subsidies to the elderly, and services within some of these apartment complexes with growing concentrations of elderly (the naturally occurring retirement communities [NORCs]) are expanding. The NORCs have a marketing advantage because residents are already in place and do not have to move.

The private-market feasibility studies, of course, ignore at least two thirds of the elderly, who are not income-qualified. For the most part, these individuals must rely on the facilities that are supported only by public and private charitable dollars. In contrast to the private market, the lack of privacy and amenities offered by these facilities dampens demand.

For example, few of the adult homes in New York City that accept SSI recipients are attractive to potential elderly clients who are still able to live in their own apartments in neighborhoods where they still have friends and where similar personal care services are available. Many adult homes, despite numbers that suggest there should be some pent-up demand, are operating at relatively low occupancy rates. According to state health department officials, those facilities were operating at about 82% of capacity statewide in 2001.

Getting the Financing

Nationally, assisted living construction project costs ranged from $111,000 to $142,000 per unit in the year 2000 (Moore 2001). The range of construction costs in New York City is about twice that national figure. In New York City, the total capital budget for construction of a one-hundred-unit assisted living facility could run between $12 million and $25 million and would be higher still in Manhattan. That total project cost includes the working capital needed to cover costs during the critical "fill-up" period between the completion of the construction or renovations and the desired stable occupancy level. The "fill-up" period marks the transition from reliance on investment sources or borrowing to self-sufficiency from the rental payments of residents to cover costs (Moore 1998).

The working capital needed to cover development, construction, and the fill-up period can come in a variety of forms and from a variety of sources. Local individual investors can provide the cash in return for an ownership stake. Sometimes local investors assume the full cost of construction and contract with an assisted living company to manage the operation. Management companies charge from 4% to as high as 8% of gross revenues for their services. Their compensation contract might also include bonus incentives for meeting occupancy targets or profit goals. A real estate investment trust (REIT) representing many investors desiring a diversified managed real estate portfolio similar to that of a stock fund can also provide a source of capital. During the boom period of development in the 1990s, REITs were a common source of capital. Alternatively, a privately held assisted living company could finance the project using internally generated funds. Although targeted rates of return are often not achieved, the eventual return on investment can be as high as 40% (Moore 2001). For an individual investor willing to take the risk and wait several years to realize a return, new assisted living new construction can be an attractive investment opportunity. A publicly traded assisted living company, as described in the previous chapter, may be able to raise capital by a stock offering. An assisted living company may also borrow money from a bank just as an individual might in acquiring a mortgage for a home.

Assisted living companies, much like the recently bankrupt Enron Corporation, sometimes cleverly concealed risks from prospective investors. Companies in the industry have practiced so-called black-box financing. In its most extreme form, it kept the start-up losses off the balance sheet while reporting the management fees accruing from the venture as income. For investors unfamiliar with the practice, the firm's financial statements often communicated an unrealistically rosy picture that helped fuel the rise in the company's stock prices. As long as the new venture worked according to plan, all the partners in such an arrangement were happy. However, problems began in 1998, when fill-up in projects began to fall behind schedule and deficits mounted. A sequence of events in early 1999 sparked an investor "black-box" panic. Assisted living stocks lost 58% of their market value between April and October 1999 (Sapphir 1999). Assisted Living Concepts, an Oregon-based firm, triggered that drop with an announcement in February of a $10 million correction in its earnings for the two previous calendar years. An independent audit for American Retirement Corporation of Nashville, which had announced plans to acquire Assisted Living Concepts for $487 million, triggered the correction. The auditors questioned the accounting practices related to Assisted Living Concepts' "black box," and as a result, American Retirement dropped its plans to acquire Assisted Living Concepts. A flurry of more than a dozen class-action lawsuits by stockholders followed. The stockholders alleged securities fraud and insider trading on the part of executives of Assisted Living Concepts. The lawyers succeeded in hammering out a consolidated $30 million settlement with Assisted Living Concepts at the end of November 2000 ("Assisted Living Concepts Settles" 2000). Assisted Living Concepts operated at a loss of more than $25 million in 2000. It had incurred similar losses in 1998 and 1999. In June 2001, industry analysts were predicting that Assisted Living Concepts would be part of a second wave of bankruptcies, this time in assisted living, that would follow the earlier wave in the publicly traded nursing home sector ("Is Time Running Out" 2001). In October 2001 Assisted Living Concepts filed for Chapter 11 bankruptcy after bond holders agreed to the reorganization plan ("Company Briefs" 2001). Investors learned from these events to take a more skeptical and conservative view of the assisted living industry. They are now more likely to insist on a large equity stake in the development by the operators and a strong track record from previous projects.

If the financing of the construction or renovation of high-income assisted living developments can be difficult at times, the financing of low-income developments is akin to the magic of spinning straw into gold. Assisted Living Concepts was the only publicly traded company to attempt to provide low-income care, and this made it vulnerable to shifts in state policy over payment. At least in the New York metropolitan area, the only way to make the numbers work so that income from operations can cover the cost of indebtedness is not to have any.

The story of the development of the deSales assisted living project, constructed on 108th Street and Fifth Avenue in Spanish Harlem, illustrates the magnitude of the challenges. The facility was developed to sustain the resurgence of the transition neighborhood and to provide care for low-income residents equivalent to that offered by private-pay assisted living developments. Each of the small apartment units in the project has a private bath and kitchen. Taking advantage of all of the available forms of state payment, the facility projected a monthly income of between $2,600 and $3,000 for each resident. According to one of the developers, this was estimated to be enough to meet the day-to-day operating costs of the facility. However, it cost more than $25 million, or about $200,000 per unit, to construct the facility. The efforts to obtain these funds and develop a credible plan to pay off debt required a complex, patchwork, Rube Goldberg process, which included predevelopment loans from the Harlem Community Development Corporation, seed money from a local hospital, a $400,000 gift from a private donor, tax-exempt bonds, the sale of tax credits to for-profit companies, deferred payments to the architectural and construction firms, a $1.2 million fifteen-year loan from the Federal Home Loan Bank that would be forgiven if the facility met its intended purpose, and the financing of the remaining $7,500 per unit by a loan at 3% interest. The development was completed and is now fully occupied, but it is struggling financially. The remarkable thing is that it was created by a local group that started with no money to invest but was somehow able to spin straw into gold.

Managing the Operations

The myriad of details involved in day-to-day operations is best left to the stories that will be told about individual facilities in the next two chapters. Two general observations suffice to provide some context for understanding these stories.

First, all of the facilities have someone, most frequently referred to as a community relations director, who is responsible for maintaining the facility's stabilized occupancy. That means outreach to providers and referral sources as well as the dissemination of promotional materials to the community. It means talking with prospective residents and their families. It means intervening at times with staff and families to forestall turnover of residents. Success at these activities assures a reliable income stream.

Second, some assisted living facilities tend to be drawn into a subtle smoke and mirrors game with their prospective customers about costs. The assisted living market is price-elastic, and the key to success is the perception of good value for the price. That may involve investment in an attractive lobby and grounds to create the image of high-end affluence. It is a myth that assisted living caters to the high-income sector in the way that gated retirement communities with million-dollar price tags do. It doesn't. In most cases, it caters to the gap between those who are eligible for public entitlements and those who can afford to pay for or who have family members who can assist with round-the-clock assistance in their own homes. Developers consciously design facilities to communicate a message that the prospective residents will, by moving in, achieve a lifelong dream of upward mobility and at the same time avoid their lifelong nightmare of becoming a ward of the state, which the most common physical design of nursing homes communicates. Developers design lobbies that look like the entranceways of mansions in exclusive neighborhoods that prospective residents during their work lives could not afford to move into. They purchase properties at prestige addresses at a premium. They dress the staff that waits on the residents' tables with the black ties and starched white shirts of the waiters in the community's most exclusive restaurants. Yet the market is competitive. Providers search for ways to trim costs, which may involve reducing staff. As much as 75% of the operating costs of a facility are labor costs. Reducing the staff and staff turnover may leave inexperienced staff stretched too thin to address the increasing needs of residents who are, indeed, inevitably aging in place. It is no easy matter to balance the tensions caused by producing the margins that define success in the eyes of owners and the financial institutions that lend money and serving the needs of residents. It is especially challenging for facilities that serve those with only public support.

The Mission

To Our Residents and Their Families We Pledge:

To enhance the lives of our residents . . .

- Encourage residents to achieve and maintain their maximum level of independent function.
- Provide choices and options, through risk management programs and other means, to meet resident's needs and encourage them to continue to be actively involved in decisions about their care needs.
- Preserve each resident's dignity and privacy.

To nurture our residents . . .
- Assess each resident's needs and reassess appropriately.
- Provide appropriate and cost-effective services.

To provide safe environments and caring, competent staff . . .
- Ensure staff have appropriate background, skills, and experience and ensure that they receive necessary training to support the services offered.

To inform residents and families about services provided . . .
- Detail services available, related costs and policies relating to charges, including any changes in charges.
- Explain thoroughly the criteria or parameters for changing the level of service, including policies relating to transfers from the residence.
- Where appropriate, provide family members access to all of the information about services and involve them in decision-making.
- Identify other services available through arrangements with the provider or independently.
- Disclose existence of financial relationships with affiliated or independent providers of ancillary services.

To Our Community We Pledge:
- To coordinate care with other providers when necessary.
- To help the public & policymakers understand assisted living.
- To maintain a responsive attitude to evolving care needs of residents and respond proactively and cooperatively with other groups to best serve the needs of residents.

(Assisted Living Federation of America 2002)

Associations try to present a united front. They often smooth over controversial views of differences among members. People in the industry talk more openly among themselves:

> I think it is important for those who have been in the industry a while and for those who are thinking of getting into to it to understand what is going on. Just so you understand my background I have one foot in the nursing home industry and the other one very firmly planted in the assisted living industry. I have been in the industry as long as Paul [Klaassen]. I was with him at the first board of directors meeting, so I've seen this evolve. I want to give a little perspective here. The assisted living revolution is a revolution. The whole concept of how to care for the elderly in America has been

turned on its ear, and I say hurray! It's a good thing, and the big winners are going to be the elderly. But now we are getting the fallout from that chaos. If we wrote the history of assisted living we could call this time period the "Age of Chaos" or "Agonizing Reappraisal." The regulators see people getting hurt in assisted living and so they say, OK, we've got to get a specific staffing ratio in order to prove that there is not enough staff. It may not be right but it can be enforced. But there are not any rules because we turned the industry on its ear. Regulators said nursing homes should take care of nursing home patients. It was a level-of-care issue. But then people like Paul and Bill Lasky and others said, "No, people should have choices." Now, nobody knows what to do. It is worse because some people in assisted living want to give care all the way down the line, because that's what choice is. But others say, "No, choice means if you get too confused or too sick, you have to leave." So ALFA and the industry is now criticized both for wanting to care for people and for wanting to throw them out! We say, "Oh gosh, they (the regulators) have not figured it out." Come on, guys, get a life. We have not figured it out ourselves! It is a chaotic mess, and until it all gets sorted out over the next five or six years, we are going to have a lot of meetings like this. ("Regulatory Trends in Assisted Living" 2001)

What is the difference between the mission of assisted living and the missions of other providers of health and long-term care services? The difference can perhaps be distilled into three promises assisted living providers would like to make to the consumer of long-term care services. They are:

1. It is your home. You should have your own private apartment. Even when your financial resources do not permit all the amenities of private apartment living, you should not have to share your private space with strangers. You should be able to lock your doors and furnish your space as you wish. Your privacy will be respected. The entire layout of the "community," its lighting fixtures, grounds, common rooms, and furniture should be the same as you would have in your own home. It should be noninstitutional and nonmedical in character.
2. You have the right to choose. It is your life, and you can choose how to live it. You may choose what you do, what services you want to receive, what you want to eat, and when you will have your meals. Your independence and autonomy will be respected. You may choose to take risks even when the service providers caution you that those risks are too great.

3. You can age in place. You can receive whatever services you need (or want) without having to move to another residence. You should never have to move again.

These three promises represent a bill of rights that drastically alters the relationship between the resident or patient and those providing care. They may be presented as strongly worded assertions or more cautious and qualified ones. In either case, they distinguish assisted living from the more traditional approaches to long-term care.

In terms of the historical context outlined in Chapter 2, proponents of assisted living advocate "outdoor relief." It is helpful to contrast the promises outlined above with the rules that typically governed poorhouses in the nineteenth century, the predecessors of the modern nursing home. For example, the rules governing residents in a Massachusetts poor farm in 1884 provide a useful benchmark:

1. A court order is required to commit inmates.
2. Inmates must rise at hour appointed by superintendent.
3. Seats are assigned in the dining room.
4. No cooking outside the kitchen.
5. Lights out at a specified time.
6. Males and females shall not associate together.
7. "Ardent Spirits" prohibited.
8. Smoking allowed only in the smoking room.
9. Permission for day-leave secured from superintendent.
10. Inmates must return before sunset.

(quoted in Manard et al. 1977, 28)

Institutional long-term care has certainly moved far from such harsh rules, but a chasm remains between the promises of assisted living providers and the current realities of long-term care. How close do specific assisted living facilities themselves come in honoring such promises?

Honoring the promises made by assisted living providers poses seemingly insurmountable challenges. How do providers assure safety and a high standard of care for residents while allowing them the freedom to take risks and have choice in the care they receive? Even if state agencies allowed assisted living facilities the necessary flexibility to keep these promises, they cannot avoid the liability issues. Liability insurers insist on controlling the risks and on meeting standards of care similar to that of other long-term care providers. Financial backers and lenders insist on liability insurance coverage. No money for the development of assisted living projects, no assisted living. Checkmate.

In essence, assisted living cannot separate itself from the mainstream of the development of safety and quality-of-care standards for other health care providers. It is foolish to pretend that it can and essential that it makes the best use of what has been learned in this process.

The Evolution of Safety and Quality-of-Care Standards for Health Care Facilities

Just as assisted living facilities are now a diverse collection of institutions lacking any common agreed-upon care standards at the beginning of the twenty-first century, so were hospitals at the beginning of the twentieth century. Charlatans abounded, building their own private "hospitals" and promoting their own special "cures." Physicians who referred a patient to a surgeon at one of these fledgling hospitals would "fee split" or, in current parlance, get a kickback for the referral. How could the public be protected? Should one rely on the market and the voluntary policing of providers or state regulation? Market forces and state regulation, in essence, took a backseat to the medical profession, and, specifically, the efforts of the American College of Surgeons to impose standards on hospitals. The Joint Commission on Accreditation of Health Care Organizations (JCAHO), predecessor of these early efforts, began in 2001 to provide a similar service to the assisted living industry. The less medically dominated Commission on Accreditation of Rehabilitation Facilities began a similar initiative in the same year. The success in achieving a degree of standardization among hospitals through the voluntary hospital standardization program, however, was largely a result of the insistence of health care insurers. Blue Cross, commercial plans, and subsequently, the Medicare and Medicaid programs, in essence, refused to pay for services in facilities that were not accredited. Hospitals that are accredited by JCAHO are eligible to receive payment under Medicare. Hospitals not accredited must be certified as meeting federal standards by the state agency that licenses and inspects facilities. They must also be certified by this same agency to receive Medicaid funds. The federal and state standards, however, are largely modeled after those of JCAHO.

Accreditation also made it easier to raise money for renovation, expansion, and replacement of facilities. Hospitals, like almost all organizations, have always adhered to the Golden Rule: those with the gold rule. The success of voluntary assisted living accreditation efforts will probably be tied to similar developments. Unless accreditation becomes a condition for payment, it is unlikely to become widely adopted.

Concern about enforcing standards of care in hospitals, however, did not truly become internalized in hospitals until 1965, when a court decision in Illinois stripped the last vestiges of charitable immunity from liability from nonprofit hospitals. Up until that time, only the outside direct provider of care could be sued for malpractice (*Darling v. Charleston Community Hospital* 1965), and hospitals had little need to carry liability insurance and no need to develop any procedures for managing risks. Nursing homes were similarly affected in the wake of this decision's impact on hospitals. But because nursing homes were not generally financed by private insurance at that time, certification was imposed on them instead by state agencies.

In retrospect, the limitations of the hospital standardization and quality assurance approach seem obvious. Efforts to improve safety were handicapped both by a reluctance to report, document, and analyze incidents that would provide a paper trail that could expose them to greater legal liability and by the focus on individual professional responsibility (blame) inevitable in any professionally dominated standardization process. The accreditation process focused on the credentials of staff and the structure of governance rather than the experiences or outcomes of patients. Reports recently released in an Institute of Medicine (IOM) study of safety and quality assurance in health care highlight the predictable limitations of such approaches to the standardization and the improvement of care (Institute of Medicine 1999; Institute of Medicine 2001). The IOM study concludes that basic safety assurance in hospitals is weakened by an atmosphere in which errors are underreported and safety is considered the responsibility of the individual professional and not a part of the design of systems of care. As a result, more than 44,000 patients die in the United States each year from easily correctable medical errors (Institute of Medicine 1999, 1). This conservative estimate makes such mistakes the eighth leading cause of death. The cost of these errors is more than $17 billion a year (Institute of Medicine 1999, 1).

Yet safety alone is but a small part of the problem. The system of health care as a whole detracts from the health, dignity, functioning, comfort, satisfaction, and resources of citizens (Institute of Medicine 2001). It falls far short of the growing expectations and needs of patients for a continuous healing relationship, control, free-flowing access to information, and seamless cooperation between providers of care. The Assisted Living Quality Coalition began an effort directed toward meeting those needs and addressing the issues of standardization in 1996 (Assisted Living Quality Coalition 1998).

The IOM report described health care as a whole as a "complex adaptive system," and the same description applies to assisted living. Unlike mechanical systems, such systems have the capacity to learn and change as a result of experience. NORCs and assisted living facilities, for example, have both done a remarkable job of adapting to the increasing needs of their residents. As with other complex adaptive systems, this has been achieved by having a common organizational purpose, motivated participants, and a few simple rules to guide their complex adaptive behavior. The following, derived by substituting *resident* for "patient" and *caregiver* for "clinician" in the ten simple rules proposed in the IOM report (Institute of Medicine 2001, 16), could well serve as guides for safety and quality improvement in assisted living:

1. Care is based on a continuous healing relationship
2. Care is customized according to resident needs and values.
3. The resident is the source of control.
4. Knowledge is shared and information flows freely.
5. Decision-making is evidence-based.
6. Safety is a system property.
7. Transparency is necessary.
8. Needs are anticipated.
9. Waste is continuously decreased.
10. Cooperation among caregivers is a priority.

Perhaps it will be possible for assisted living in the twenty-first century to leapfrog, rather than simply repeat, the twentieth-century history of hospital standardization and quality improvement and the licensure and inspection process for nursing homes that followed in its wake.

The business of assisted living blends real estate development and health care. It operates in the gray area between housing and health services, where the distinctive approaches of these two sectors often collide. The mission of assisted living sets it at odds with the concerns about safety and quality of care in traditional health settings. It argues for the same choice, autonomy, and ability to take risks that one has in one's own home. Yet an even more fundamental conflict dwarfs these. It is embedded in the recurring tensions in the history of care described in Chapter 2—the role of government, institutional care, and control. In essence, the larger conflict involves a choice between class and community. Should care for the frail elderly, like other goods and services, be organized by the market, according to people's ability to pay? Should it be a privilege of the few or a universal right?

In the next chapter I address how conflicts over margin and mission affect five facilities that care for those who can afford to pay for the privilege. In the chapter after that, I contrast these stories with the experiences of caregivers, administrators, and residences of five facilities that care for those who can't afford such privileged care. I explore the implications of the choices these facilities have made between margin, mission, class, and community. Perhaps then our own choices will be clearer.

5
Private-Pay Assisted Living

The organization of health and social services in the United States changed in the twentieth century. In 1900, hospitals, county homes, and other institutions cared almost exclusively for the indigent. Nursing students, as a part of their training, provided much of the direct care. Most nurses left these institutions after graduation to serve as private-duty nurses in the homes of families that needed and could afford their services. Most of a physician's private practice involved making house calls and caring for patients in their own homes. As medical advances progressed, hospitals became the preferred site of care, not the last resort of the destitute. This shift culminated with the integration of private-pay and indigent patients after the implementation of Medicare and Medicaid.

The emergence of private-market assisted living at the end of the twentieth century began to swing the pendulum back in the opposite direction. This chapter explores the potential implications of this swing through five case studies of facilities that cater to the private-pay market. National for-profit chains operate two of them, two are operated by nonprofits, and one is owner-operated. Two are in urban locations and three in suburban locations. While facilities like these could be located anywhere in the United States, their licensure status reflects the distinctive laws of New York State. Two are licensed as adult homes, one as enriched housing, and two are unlicensed. All five meet the broad definition of assisted living facilities, as they "provide or arrange for assisted living services such as personal care services or help with activities of daily living such as bathing, dressing and toileting" (Nursing Home Community Coalition 2000, 1). I will use the general framework developed in the previous chapter, describing first the business strategy and then the way each has addressed the distinctive demands that assisted living services face. The facilities described in this chapter are identified by the following pseudonyms:

1. Harbor View: A licensed private-pay, owner-operated adult home in New York City.
2. Residential Suites: An unlicensed private-pay proprietary facility in New York City, locally owned but operated by an assisted living management company.
3. Suburban Manor: An unlicensed private-pay facility in suburban New York owned and operated by a publicly traded chain.
4. Health Campus Village: A licensed private-pay enriched housing facility in Upstate New York owned and operated as part of a nonprofit hospital-developed integrated delivery system.
5. Shady Oaks: A licensed private-pay, nonprofit adult home in suburban New York.

At the end of the chapter I will explore the question of the longer-term impact of the development of exclusively private-pay assisted living such as these five.

Harbor View

Business Strategy

MARKET NICHE

Harbor View is a licensed adult home catering to private clientele that, according to its brochure, "offers a luxurious lifestyle in a secure and caring environment." The facility has almost two hundred residents. It is a family-owned operation that opened about thirty years ago in the midst of the darkening storm of scandals that were to engulf the city's nursing home industry. The grandfather of the family started the business by opening a nursing home in a tight-knit ethnic community. The business now includes nursing homes as well as this assisted living facility. The facility receives high marks from state regulators. It has a solid reputation in the community. Among peers in the business, it has a reputation for innovation in providing high-quality care for the frail elderly. The family member who currently serves as the administrator handles the day-to-day operations with humor, energy, and insight. There is little turnover of employees, and all seem enveloped in a large extended family that extends to the residents and their families. The location offers residents stunning views, which give the impression of a resort hotel.

Careful monitoring of operating margins and an elegant adaptation to private and public sources of income for this business result in a profitable operation. The facility will not accept or keep residents who cannot pay its private rates. They have, however, on occasion, accepted residents whose families have made up the difference between the facility's rate and the Supplemental Security Income (SSI) rate.

The facility recently opened an adult day care center whose clientele are almost exclusively Medicaid recipients, for whom the facility receives approximately $100 per day per client. According to the administrator, the opening of this program was, in part, an effort to respond to community pressure to provide care to low-income members of the community. It is also profitable. Setting up the adult day care center also added value to the services that could be provided to the private-paying residents. The development of the space in the facility for the adult day care center created an attractive physical and occupational therapy room with all the appropriate and most up-to-date equipment. The facility's private residents have access to physical therapy and rehabilitation treatment rooms in the afternoons after the day care clients leave, free of charge. The only condition is that their physician prescribe the care. Some of the private residents receive Medicare payments for physical and occupational therapy provided by a home health agency, but such care does not normally provide access to such often-essential equipment. Thus the public-pay patients help subsidize free care for the private-pay residents. In addition, the business has no qualms about admitting first-day-eligible Medicaid recipients to its nursing homes.

Harbor View occupies a dominant and, until recently, uncontested position in its local market area. "We have no competition. We don't believe in it. We will work with anyone. There is plenty of need for these kind of services," the administrator said, and the community relations director echoed the same sentiments. However, they have some concern about the newly built facilities constructed by national chains in the surrounding area, which now provide similarly attractive options for those who can pay private rates. In addition, according to the administrator, more troubling recent competition is now coming from the "lower-class nursing homes and rehabilitation centers." Those are the ones that cannot fill their beds as a result of recent overall declines in occupancy and have begun to compete for private-pay residents.

Referrals are largely word of mouth. "We live and die by word of mouth," the administrator said. The overwhelming preponderance of residents comes from the same zip code as the facility, about 85%. Indeed, several residents whom we talked with later in a focus group were longtime neighbors and actually recalled the construction of the facility. There is also some reverse migration from Florida to be near children. About 60% of current admissions come directly from hospitals or nursing homes, and the remainder from private homes. Occupancy used to average almost 100%. In 1999, however, demand dropped and occupancy dipped to 90%, in part as a result of the new competition from facilities opened by national chains in the area. Occupancy has since rebounded and now stands at around 95%. In contrast, other facilities in the market area, according to the facility's administrator, are experiencing a drop to 80–85%. In a tacit acknowledgment of the growing competition to fill private beds, the facility has begun to accept individuals with walkers. In terms of discharges and admissions, the facility continues to work with all the local voluntary hospitals in the area. The community relations director explained, "I meet with all the predictable sources: the hospital discharge planners and social workers. I also go to the less obvious sources: hairdressers and manicurists. We target both the prospective resident and the adult children. We are seeing significantly more cognitive impairment and walkers on admission."

Not to be undone by more recent competition, the business is currently renovating space for an Alzheimer's care unit. The administrator envisions occupancy of most of the spaces in the unit being internally generated from the existing population of residents. In addition, a luxurious unlicensed assisted living facility, complete with a multistory atrium and swimming pool, will soon be constructed. "It will be unlicensed because you can't get licensed beds, or at least it takes forever," the administrator said.

FINANCES

The cost of care at Harbor View could exhaust the ability of some residents and families to pay for it. Monthly rates range from $1,800 for semi-private accommodations to $7,000 for two-room suites with a view in the luxury wing. Residents who need basic personal care (dressing, bathing, being brought to meals, etc.) may purchase this care plan for an additional $175 per week. The charge is more for incontinence care, walks, and hourly checks. All of those personal care services are subcontracted with an outside home health agency. In addition to the $175-per-week care plan, the home health agency provides one-on-one care with an aide for twelve hours a day for $1,000 a week and for twenty-four hours a day for $1,225 per week plus the bed rate for the aide. That could bring the overall cost of care for an individual requiring twenty-four-hour supervision to over $100,000 per year. Residents can pay for personal care attendants around the clock either through the agency that the facility subcontracts with or directly with agencies or individuals of their own choosing.

Yet Harbor View does no formal screening of applicants to determine their ability to pay. The administrator explained, "We ask for absolutely nothing in terms of financial documentation, but the financial obligations that will be incurred are explained, and we advise applicants and families likely to exhaust their resources to look elsewhere. An admission here is neither in their best interest or ours." The administrator had a dim view of some of the pricing policies of other facilities. "We are familiar with what everyone else does in pricing various services, but we don't believe we should nickel-and-dime people to death. Families resent this." According to the administrator, the self-selection process in choosing a facility has made dealing with residents who exhaust their ability to pay a very rare occurrence. "If a family runs out of money, we will advise. We have never had to throw out a resident," he said. Indeed, the exhaustion of residents' assets at Harbor View often triggers discharges as first-day-eligible Medicaid admissions to one of its nursing homes.

If a resident is not eligible for Medicaid, before they run out of funds, "we get the family together and work with them," the administrator explained. "I go through the numbers with people, and if it looks like they are not going to have enough, I give them the names of other facilities. I don't refuse, but I explain to them that it's not fair to their relative." The community relations director was more troubled by the front end of the affordability problem. "It kills me to tell people to look elsewhere who don't have the money," she said. "I go to people's homes, and I've seen everything. Mostly it's the loneliness that brings them here. Times have changed, and we have two-job households and the kids can't have mom at home now."

Yet this firmness pays off, as evidenced by the facility's strong financial track record. Getting financing for expansion is not a major problem. The strong financial track record and the equity that the owners can invest will raise no red flags for potential creditors.

MANAGING OPERATIONS

The most interesting thing about the operation of this facility is how it has adapted to its changing staffing needs. When the facility opened thirty years ago, it was in part an attractive haven for empty-nest singles. Staff functioned more the way they would in any resort hotel. Over time, staff roles changed, while the ambiance of a resort hotel was maintained. The receptionists now act as a nerve center, coordinating the care of residents. They schedule doctor appointments, make sure residents get to their appointments, and assist residents with medications. The waiters and waitresses also receive personal care training and monitor the eating habits of residents, encouraging and guiding them regarding good nutrition. The maitre d' periodically weighs residents before meals and keeps track of those who do not show. Calls are made to the rooms of no-shows to encourage attendance. If persuasion fails, food is sent to the room and caregivers are alerted. The room attendants, or housekeepers, are also trained as personal care aides, with one assigned to each floor of thirty to forty units. They monitor various problems such as incontinence, bleeding, and possible adverse reactions to medications. They are, in effect, almost doubling as floor nurses. Those responsibilities appear to have evolved from the regular monthly meetings of department heads, which have the structure of an interdisciplinary problem-solving team. A year ago, weekly interdisciplinary meetings for all those providing direct care were added, focusing on the needs of individual residents. Two licensed home health agencies provide care to residents. One provides the personal care under subcontract with the facility. The other provides Medicare-reimbursed skilled services to residents. That agency simply rents space from the facility and bills separately.

The facility has been inventive in cutting through red tape, which has facilitated the access of residents to services that they feel residents need. It was recently approved as a limited-licensed home health agency. Licensing as an on-site home health agency that would be qualified to receive Medicare funds involves too much red tape. A limited-license home health agency enables the facility to hire a licensed nurse to administer the medications. A licensed adult home cannot hire a nurse to do that. The home is allowed only to "assist" with medications. A nurse, however, cannot "assist" but can only "administer." A nurse hired by the limited-licensed home health agency is, in effect, part of the facility, but it creates the necessary fiction to permit the nurse to administer medications. (Should we wonder why so many elderly people have trouble finding their way through the health and social service system that is supposed to be there to help them?)

Responding to the Demands of Assisted Living
A HOME, CHOICE, AND A PLACE TO GROW OLD

The higher-priced accommodations at Harbor View are attractive private apartments with spectacular views. "It's like a hotel. The difference is that you don't have quite the independence, but you don't have to fend for yourself as you would in your own home," one resident explained. "Not wanting to cook, clean, or be alone" was the motivation for several of the women residents we talked with. "I didn't like to be at home. I wanted to be with people," one said. One woman came for the two-week trial and it was then suggested that she at least "stick around for the Jewish holidays." That was almost ten year ago. For most of the residents, however, a medical crises or loss of spouse was the precipitating event that resulted in relocation to Harbor View.

Some of the residents we talked with shared an apartment with another resident. While most began the session talking about how nice it was to have a roommate and how reassuring it was not to be alone, it later became clear that most had begun their residency with private rooms and that the major factor causing the change to a double room was affordability. One was quite angry and defensive about her move to a double room. When asked for the reason for the shift to double rooms, one replied, "Come on, didn't you go to college?" The implication was that the answer was obvious and it was not nice to ask.

In some respects, what makes assisted living different from living at home has nothing to do with the facility itself. The difference is the change in the relationship it signifies with one's children. The children are now more in charge, and both parties resist the change. "When they bring their parents into a facility like this, they need to bring themselves as well. You're moving not just things, you're losing power," the care coordinator says. "They say, 'This is not my mom,' but it is, and they need to understand the transition. They need to be sensitive, not just to cut the visit short if their mother is getting upset. They need to put themselves in their parents' shoes and give them a little extra time. We send letters out each month to family members about what their relative is doing, but we only get a handful of responses back." Most children have difficulty acknowledging the changes: "'I don't want my mother to wear

Pampers,' one tells us. Some have an attitude toward the aides. Sometimes they complain about the way we dress them when the family supplies the clothes for them."

In some respects, residents have much the same freedom they would have in their own homes. The administrator said, "The law says I have no choice. We notify and document, trying to change the care plan to accommodate the residents' wishes. I let residents come and go as they wish, and unfortunately, when they don't come home at night, I search the neighborhood. We do care management and document." Those providing the direct day-to-day care were less willing to allow their charges such freedom. One expressed a strong unwillingness to accede to a resident's decision if she judged it as too risky: "You can't do it, not on my shift. I care too much about you." While sexual relationships are viewed as a private matter, the facility did intervene in one case. "She was not capable of understanding," a staff member explained. "She thought that every male person was her husband. We brought the family in and stopped it."

Almost half the residents show up at the resident council's monthly meetings. The "council" has no officers or role in decision making but serves simply as a forum for providing residents information about planned changes and getting feedback. However, the facility appears to try hard to be responsive to the concerns aired by residents.

Those who can afford to pay for the additional services can age in place in this facility. "We will provide any level of care that isn't specifically prohibited," the administrator says. The administrator acknowledged that there are limits, such as when a resident cannot feed or be assisted in feeding by an aide, has recurring falls, or becomes a danger to himself or others.

There has been, in effect, considerable aging in place. When the facility first opened, many residents had their own cars, and some had full-time jobs. Now the downstairs hallways with narrower corridors (the upper-floor corridors and doors are more spacious, built to nursing home standards) are congested with walkers. This is a result of both the aging in place of the facility's longer-term residents and a change in the nature of its newer admissions.

The administrator adds, "The growing number of cognitively impaired has also impinged on the quality of life of other residents, and we have had complaints. We thought we'd have the same problem with walkers. The way I approached the resident councils was to say, 'Thank

God I don't need a walker. If I needed a walker, would you be willing to let me stay?' I explained the planned change in policies and asked for their feedback. It was a matter of presentation. If I had simply sent out a memo on stationery, we would have had a lot of complaints."

The thirty-unit Alzheimer floor is being developed for the kind of aging in place that is inappropriate for an adult home where residents are free to come and go as they please. Current residents with Alzheimer's can probably fill the unit. "It is a major problem, a medical one, and the creation of the unit was mostly internally motivated both in terms of the needs of the residents and the complaints of other residents," the administrator says. Approximately 30% of current residents have some degree of cognitive impairment.

The residents themselves were ambivalent about the notion of aging in place. They found residents with Alzheimer's difficult to be around. "They interfere with the games, they talk, and some are very depressing to be around. Some have bad manners. It affects the quality of life here," one resident said. Some indicated that they wouldn't want to be at the facility if they got sicker. Others like the idea of having a companion and staying put.

ASSURING SAFETY AND HIGH STANDARDS OF CARE

Assisted living facilities could have much more flexibility with regard to who is cared for and how, if they were given an option. A recent legislative proposal by New York's governor would allow facilities simply to "register" rather than comply with the more detailed standards of licensure. Asked which he would choose if given the option, the administrator said, "I would pick registration. Inspectors have to find problems. Then it goes on my record. It is a process that only focuses on the negatives. Let them come in and say, 'What have you done to improve the quality?' If the regulations enhance attractiveness, consumer acceptance, I'm for them. For most facilities, if you give them the money to do a good job, they will do it, and overall it will cost one third less. Why does a newspaper find serious problems and not the inspectors?"

The key to high-quality care, acknowledged by the administrator, care coordinators, and residents, is the quality of the direct care staff. The quality of the direct care staff is hard to document by an external inspection process but was clearly present in this facility. There is very little staff turnover. Most have worked for the facility for many years.

They seem to know instinctively how to work with residents and form strong personal bonds with them. One personal care aide that exuded these qualities said, "The residents are sicker, and more need walkers now. They need more assistance, but I know how to work with them. The male residents pat my behind, and I tell them, 'If I get pregnant, you'll be responsible!' What else can you do? You have to turn it into something light and fun. When you are away for two days, they miss you. Even when the mind is not always there, they know you and know who is there. One told me, 'What are you doing here, you should be a psychiatrist!' I was with this one resident for many years. One day while I was washing her, she turned around and said, 'I wish you could have been my daughter!' She hugged me and died on my shoulder. I was hysterical and I cried and cried for hours."

Yet the same aides acknowledge the discrepancy between their own social and financial circumstances and those they care for. "You are going to be there someday and whatever you do in life, one day somebody is going to do for you," one said. "They are a mirror. You can see what one day you are going to be. I want the same care I am giving, but I'll never be able to afford it. The best I can expect is a space in the parking lot!" Identification and empathy is the simple rule governing their approach to caring for residents. Yet their income and what it would entitle them to when they face similar circumstances in old age strains at their essential bond with the residents.

Residential Suites

Business Strategy

MARKET NICHE

Residential Suites is an unlicensed assisted living facility locally owned but managed by a national for-profit chain. Originally a hotel, it is clearly visible from one of the major arteries leading from the suburbs into New York City. The hotel was completely renovated three years ago to a two-hundred-unit assisted living complex. In its brief history, the facility has undergone three changes in management firms.

The lower level provides attractive dining areas, and the first floor includes a large lounge for afternoon social activities, an auditorium for bingo and exercise activities, and a large enclosed patio area for barbecues and other gatherings. The first floor appears cramped because of a high degree of participation of residents in activities. The level of participation is attributable the relatively good health of the residents and the rich activities programs offered. The first floor also provides office space for a home health agency, a visiting nurse practitioner, dentists, and physicians who bill Medicare on a fee-for-service basis. The upper floors house apartment units. One wing of the second floor houses an Alzheimer's unit. The design is attractive and well thought-out.

The large sign on top of the facility has apparently been useful in attracting residents. Commuting adult children pass the sign and occasionally some stop by to check it out for one of their parents. Nevertheless, the facility has struggled to break even financially. It took almost two and a half years to fill. Six months after it opened, only fifty of its almost two hundred units were rented. Only recently did it reach 95% occupancy and begin turning a profit. The assessment of the local owner is that the former management companies tried to grow too fast and were out of touch with the local market.

Residential Suites competes with services and amenities similar to those of other facilities in the area but at a lower price. Its price, however, is still out of reach of the elderly residents in its immediate area. Its new residents come from a broader geographic area, either directly from home or from rehabilitation facilities. There are few direct placements from hospitals, and no one is initially admitted with extensive nursing and medical needs. (At least that is assumed by the facility, since there is no medical evaluation prior to admission.) The home health agency does an assessment of new residents after they have been admitted. Residential Suites presents itself as a residential hotel for seniors with an array of personal care and health services available to residents on site for those who wish to purchase them.

FINANCING

The facility accepts only private-fee-paying residents. Residents who run out of funds are assisted in seeking other care. The monthly fee ranges from $1,600 for a shared unit to $3,500 for one of the larger single-occupancy suites. This fee includes room and board, housekeeping, twenty-four-hour security, and the activities program. The home health agency bills on a private-fee basis, and none of its services are reimbursable by Medicare or Medicaid. The nurse practitioner and physician from a local hospital and some other medical professionals accept Medicare.

The fees for various personal care services provided by the home health agency range from $250 a month for occasional assistance with baths, dressing, and ambulation to a combined charge of more than $5,000 a month for the care of dementia residents.

The lack of any systematic assessment or review of financial assets prior to admission creates uncertainty about whether residents will get the care they need. The management company has applied for a home health agency license, in part because of the need for greater coordination and in part because this is the most profitable part of the operation. Residents, on the other hand, complained that some of the neighbors really need more care than they were getting and some needed to be on the dementia unit. Facility administrators and the home health agency supervisor both acknowledged situations when residents were assisted without charge. Some residents are getting the assistance that they need even when they or their families chose not to purchase it or could not afford it. Caregivers invent solutions and try to overcome the limitations of the way the facility is organized.

OPERATIONS

In theory, the owner and the firms that have been responsible for managing the facility have no direct responsibility for the direct care provided to residents. The fiction is that as an unlicensed facility it provides no direct health or personal care to residents. That is the responsibility of the on-site licensed home health agency. Residents have a separate service agreement with the home health agency and are charged separately. Staff, however, know what is going on informally between the home health agency and residential sides of the operation. The cost of the two recreational aides on the Alzheimer's unit is covered by the residential side of the operation but overlaps with the direct care provided by the home health service side of the operation. There are also weekly meetings that combine the supervisors of both components so that information about residents is shared.

The most remarkable thing about the facility, however, is how smoothly the day-to-day operations function and how insulated they are from these confusing operational fictions and management turmoil. Despite the changes in management, the same staff, supervisors, and aides continue to provide the care. The staff has gone about doing what needs to be done, and residents go about getting what they need. The stability also reflects the ability of the relatively low-paid and not formally trained staff just to do what makes sense to them.

Responding to the Demands of Assisted Living
A HOME, CHOICE, AND A PLACE TO GROW OLD

Residential Suites' attractive first-floor lounges bubble with activity. Several groups chat and drink tea in the snack area; an exercise class is in progress in the room where a bingo session will soon follow. Private and spacious efficiency and one- and two-bedroom apartments occupy the floors above. Two dining rooms, one formal and one more informal, both with fresh flowers on the tables, offer a variety of menu choices to residents. The administrator says she tells prospective residents, "This is your apartment, and you can live here for the rest of your life." In many ways that is a fair assessment. About 30% of the residents are currently receiving care from the home health agency. The facility, however, reserves the right to ask residents to leave whom they believe they can't care for adequately or who refuse the additional care that the home health agency feels is essential.

Unlike Harbor View, however, the surrounding community is alien territory for residents, and none come from the immediate area. The site served as an appropriate spot for a hotel but not as a place well integrated into a local community. Some of the residents are unhappy about being dislocated and isolated from old friends and neighborhoods.

Both residents and staff acknowledge that, in the end, there is nothing the staff can do to prevent residents from subjecting themselves to serious risks. Residents may come and go as they like, eat what they like, etc. The management of care in the facility places clear limits on the ability of staff to control the behavior of residents.

There is a resident council that has an executive committee but no officers because no one wants the titles. The activities director convenes and conducts the meetings. The members of the executive committee see their role as similar to that of a ward or block captain in a neighborhood. Residents might go to them if they have a problem that needs to be addressed by management. It sounds like a good idea, but the residents with whom we talked were unaware of the council or who was on it.

In theory, the services available at extra cost allow an individual to age in place, which honors the promise of an apartment where one can remain for the rest of his or her life. Yet, as the administrator acknowledged, if a resident is no longer able to participate in the activities programs or is no longer able to eat or ambulate independently, the quality-of-life argument for remaining at the facility becomes weaker. Residents who are able to participate in activities are not happy with the aging that is taking place. As one observed, "We don't want to turn the mirror around and look at ourselves." Some specifically chose the facility because they wanted to be around more life and liveliness and not around so many old people. Successful aging in place perhaps requires not only additional services but the acceptance and compassionate involvement of other residents.

ASSURING SAFETY AND HIGH STANDARDS OF CARE

In many respects Residential Suites functions more like a naturally occurring retirement community than a health facility. It works remarkably well, given the seemingly ad hoc and informal manner in which the needs of residents are met. The home health agency staff chips in and provides needed care for residents even when there is no contractual relationship and no payment for their help. There is even one resident receiving care in the Alzheimer's unit who is not formally a patient of the home health agency.

Although there are weekly meetings between the supervisors of the home health agency and the facility's staffs, there is no real case management. Things just happen. One would feel more comfortable about such a flexible, seat-of-the-pants approach if it were not for the limited training and inexperience of most of the staff.

Suburban Manor

Business Strategy

MARKET NICHE

A national chain recently constructed Suburban Manor, an unlicensed facility in an affluent suburban community. It is a beautifully designed building that houses about one hundred residents. The lower floors have units for residents who are cognitively in tact or have slight cognitive impairments. The upper floor has units for the residents with dementia. All of the residents have private apartments that range from studio apartments to suites. Meals are served restaurant style. About 50% of the square footage of the complex is devoted to attractive common areas in an attempt to encourage socialization. The layout gives a favorable first impression to adult children who may be exploring options for their aging parents. Considerable thought has gone into the overall design, operational policies, and procedures. The corporation has, in fact, standardized design and operations.

The national chain also applies careful planning to selecting its locations, and at least in this case it has paid off. The facility filled in less than one hundred days after its opening, almost three months ahead of schedule, and it now operates at over 95% occupancy. In selecting sites, the firm looks for a concentration of households headed by persons between the ages of forty-five and sixty and with household incomes over $75,000. The firm considers adult children of aging parents its customers. The daughters are the main targets. The parent almost never makes the decision on his or her own and usually only agrees after succumbing to the pressures of the adult children.

Suburban Manor has carved out a strong position in the local market. On the one hand, it caters effectively to the concerns of adult children by providing an attractive, safe environment near where they live. The adult children cannot be accused (or accuse themselves) of committing their parents to an institution. In other words, the facility, or "community" as the operators would prefer to describe it, is not the dreaded nursing home. Almost half of the residents have returned from Florida or other retirement resort locations to be closer to their adult children.

On the other hand, Suburban Manor is designed and staffed to provide care for residents that other residential facilities would not able to provide. Suburban Manor provides care for incontinence and cognitive impairment that most retirement housing complexes would be unwilling to give. The managing company appears committed to allowing residents to age in place. The facility will keep anyone except those who are medically unstable or who require IVs, tubes, or vents or are on diets that need careful monitoring, such as severe diabetics, and anyone who is a danger to himself or others. Indeed, some of their referrals come from competitors who are either unwilling to accept or wish to discharge residents with problems. The managing company's major local competition comes from a few high-end licensed adult homes in the area. Referrals come from many sources, including hospital discharge planners and rehabilitation centers. As with other facilities, the basic approach of the community relations director is to become involved in the community and build relationships.

Although Suburban Manor has been essentially fully occupied almost since its opening, it expects increasing difficulty in maintaining full occupancy as other new assisted living facilities begin to open. When there was a dip in occupancy during the winter, the community relations director explored the possibility of admitting a resident with a Foley catheter, but the nurse in charge of overseeing resident health care rejected that possibility.

FINANCING

If residents run out of money, they are discharged. The facility does not ask for any financial information before admitting residents. The financial condition of the applicant, however, is read in the body language of the adult children when payments arrangements are explained. It is an informal process, but sufficient to ensure that most residents have enough resources to sustain the costs incurred as a resident in the facility for at least five years. Usually one of the adult children is the responsible party and signs the contract between the prospective resident and the managing company. Suburban Manor charges between $2,500 and $5,000 per month for a resident's apartment, meals, and activities. Anything else is extra. Personal care packages range from $23 a day to $65 a day depending on the number of hours of personal care required per day. Administration of medication costs $8 a day for two administrations. Some residents expressed irritation about everything costing extra. One resident was annoyed to receive a large bill when all she needed was help with dressing for only two days and transportation by van to a doctor. For a resident with substantial personal care needs, the "extra" costs could amount to $50,000 per year or more.

OPERATIONS

The managing company operates its own licensed home health agency, and all of the on-site care managers and personal care workers are hired by the home health agency. Among other staff there is none of the specialization typically seen in a hospital. Workers are expected to function universally and have job descriptions that, broken down into components, amount to the same functions as those performed by a mother for her child. There is a conscious attempt not to recruit individuals with experience working in nursing homes or other health-related settings for positions with either the home health agency or the facility staff. "Give me a lump of clay with a heart that I can mold rather than a nursing home aide," the director says. The company looks for people who want a second family and try to make the work fun, if not excessively remunerative. When it first opened, the facility hired seventy-five persons but interviewed almost twenty-five hundred.

At full occupancy and with its reasonably frugal approach to staffing, this facility has more than met the company's expectations for profitability.

Responding to the Demands of Assisted Living

A HOME, CHOICE, AND A PLACE TO GROW OLD

The newly constructed facility has the look and feel of a home. Its porches with rockers and its high-ceiling entrance area mix allusions to early nineteenth-century architectural style and that of modern, high-end condominium development. The property is attractively landscaped with gardens. The interior is full of light and immaculately clean. The staff know the residents by name and engage in lighthearted banter with them. Residents have the option of private or "companion" suites, which typically are occupied by couples. Residents furnish their own apartments.

Residents can self-medicate, choose their own seating for meals, smoke in the smoking room, and entertain visitors at any time. They can even have overnight guests. Residents get up when they like and select the food they want from a menu. There are two mealtime seatings. All units can be locked from the inside.

"We respect their privacy," an administrator said. Yet small erosions of that privacy slip by. The records of residents are stored with their names visible at the nurses' station where the residents see their physicians. The "advanced directives" and medication symbols on the spines are visible for all.

The residents we talked with included a couple whose son and daughter were concerned about their living far away in Florida and found the place for them. Another who had been living alone after the death of her husband had fallen several times and did not want to be in her house alone. Most chose the facility, or had it chosen for them, because it is near their adult children. One woman, who has difficulty walking, does not want to live with her children. Her daughter picked out the facility. She likes the facility because it is near her daughter's home, and her grandchildren and their dog can visit.

The facility provides a rich variety of trips, activities, in-house movies, and discussion groups for residents to choose from. Friends and family visit frequently. Some residents volunteer at the school next door. The facility organizes shopping trips, weekly trips to a restaurant, and visits to the local library. "They pay the bills," as one staff member observed. The facility's care plans are individualized and based on records about individuals' experiences and the activities that they enjoy.

Yet for most residents, it is not home. "It's a much smaller space, an apartment, not a home. It has an elevator, which I don't like," said one. Another complained, "I needed care, but I didn't expect so much added cost, and I did not expect residents to be so sick, so confused. It is like a nursing home, and residents fall asleep in wheelchairs in the front." Another was depressed by the isolation she felt. "I wanted intellectual activities," she said. "I didn't want to be a burden on family but didn't expect so many feeble persons. I can't speak to many people here, and I'm upset about all the extra costs. They are concentrating on Alzheimer's. They put them [Alzheimer's patients] in with us if they are at the beginning [stages of the disease]." Some find the new constraints of community living difficult to adjust to: "This is a big step. We gave up our independence; we live near our children, but they are busy, and we now have to live by rules. The meals are at specific times, even if there are two seatings. You can't go out and do what you want when you want to. You can have guests, but you must tell them twenty-four hours in advance. Transportation is a big problem. We were told there was a van, and there is one, but it cannot be used whenever we want. Residents want to go to more places."

Residents meet every month with the director, the activities director, and the food coordinator. This is not a council or in any way a form of governance. The purpose of the meetings is to allow the residents to complain and be heard. Corporate policy of the chain requires these meetings, and like most aspects of the home, from menu planning to décor, the meetings are planned centrally and uniformly across facilities.

The residents express a sense of loss of control and power over their lives, which are now in the hands not only of the facility but also of their children. "I complained about food, but they didn't listen. I had my son complain, and they made changes," one resident observed. One of the male residents said, "The only way they can really punish us is to call our children when we are bad. They snitch on you!" Their biggest fear, and perhaps the ultimate threat, is being shipped to the Alzheimer's unit on the top floor. In spite of the euphemistic name and amenities of this section of the facility, residents attach the same fear and same stigma to it as people once did to the back ward of a state psychiatric hospital.

While the staff acknowledge the importance of choice for residents, they have an understandable reluctance to allow more risky choices. There is no process for negotiating formal risk contracts. Staff members work hard informally to persuade residents not to take risks they are uncomfortable with. They often call the family if a resident takes risks. However, some risk-taking is tolerated, such as walking down the stairs and drinking in the rooms. When pressed, staff members acknowledged that they cannot allow residents to do things that might hurt them. "When residents choose to do things unsafe, I would say no," said one. "I would persuade, reassure. I would be afraid something might happen. I would ask the family what they want."

The facility works hard to enable residents to age in place and to honor its commitment to the residents and their families not to put them through the emotionally wrenching process of having to move again. An estimated 85% of admissions will be able to remain until death. The current residents include some who are independent and live at the facility only because they need a home or because their children are worried about their ability to manage independently. On the other hand, 50% are incontinent, and few of these can self-manage their incontinence. For these residents, the facility offers an incontinence program that seems to work well. In spite of the high proportion of residents who are incontinent, there is no odor in the facility. They have recently instituted a two-person transfer service for residents who need it. They will not keep someone who needs a Hoyer lift or requires three people to be lifted.

Thirty percent of the residents have dementia. If residents become sufficiently cognitively impaired, they will be transferred to the Alzheimer's unit on a separate floor, with controlled access and more direct care. Part of the challenge of providing for aging in place, which this facility seems strongly committed to addressing, is the resistance and denial of the adult children who find it hard to accept the decline of their parent. Like the residents themselves, the families resist transferring a relative to the dementia unit. Another challenge of allowing residents to age in place is fostering acceptance by other residents. As one observed, "We don't want to be with cognitively impaired residents. I have no problem with those with physical disabilities, except we do not like it that it looks like a nursing home. You see residents sleeping and falling out of their chairs." One resident captured the tension in the overlap between the medical and social model that this facility straddles when he said, "You can stay as long as you live unless you need nursing care. I wish they had an infirmary for acute issues. There is no doctor here. They immediately call 911."

ASSURING SAFETY AND HIGH STANDARDS OF CARE

Much of what Suburban Manor does is consistent with the simple rules proposed by the Institute of Medicine (IOM) report on closing the quality chasm summarized in the previous chapter. There is a conscious effort to make everything transparent to the family and the residents, down to the forms and contracts. Care is individualized, and the family, if not the resident, is clearly in control. A good deal of thought has gone into designing systems to reduce medication errors and risks associated with events such as falls. Medication is dispensed by LPNs, and they use the same medication carts used in nursing homes. Physicians must write prescriptions for all medications, even the over-the-counter ones. Only a few residents self-medicate. The facility has programs to address the most common problems, after first checking to ensure that the condition is not the result of medication. The incontinence program includes training for the cognitively intact. A physical therapist works with residents who have fallen or have walking problems. There is a weekly review of the care plan for each resident, and there are weekly meetings with the personal care aides to discuss the problems that have come up. The facility has gone farther in organizing care and anticipating the needs of residents than any of the other facilities we visited.

The administrator of this facility would prefer registration to licensure as a form of state oversight. He is afraid that licensure might restrict the facility's ability to admit or care for residents aging in place, which the organization views as an important part of its mission. The nursing director was less persuaded of the appropriateness of registration.

Suburban Manor is, however, not without the staffing problems facilities commonly face in trying to assure safety and high-quality care for residents. Caregivers work short-staffed if someone calls in sick. The most difficult part of their job is when residents get upset or angry. "My English is not good, and it's hard when residents get depressed and cry that nobody loves them—I love them," said one. The staff also become attached to residents and find it hard to deal with their decline. The dementia floor poses particular burdens on the staff. Problems arise from residents dying or deteriorating. It's traumatic for the unit. They do memorial services. They know that what works today may not work tomorrow. There is a grieving process attached to the decline of residents on the unit.

The facility pays personal care aides $9.00 to $9.50 an hour. Although the director did not acknowledge any problem in getting staff, the facility holds interviews every Tuesday afternoon, and all the personal care aides we interviewed were new. It is not clear that the facility will succeed in attracting and retaining staff in the way Harbor View has done, particularly with the mix of residents moving toward an overlap with typical nursing home patients. All these problems seem to be moderated by what the aides feel is good communication with the director.

The aides freely express their views about working for the facility. One aide likes the fact that, unlike in nursing homes, residents have everything they need in their rooms. A lead care manager helps as shifts change, providing verbal and written tips and instructions to the oncoming shift. "There is a buddy system here," one aide explained. "We are given a list of care managers to call if we cannot come in. We change shifts for each other." Both care managers love working at the facility and like the staff. "It's like having a second home," one of them said.

The residents indicated that, other than the possibility of no longer being able to afford the facility's costs, the major reason they would leave is that if current staff members leave, they may be replaced by others who are not as wonderful as the staff they have now. The residents feel that the facility is a "safe" place. They feel secure, and that is important to them. For the residents, the direct care providers are key to creating that sense of security.

Health Campus Village

The Business Strategy

MARKET NICHE

Health Campus Village is a recent addition to a hospital-developed integrated delivery system. It is located on a spacious suburban hospital campus. Health Campus Village is a licensed enriched housing facility that provides meals and personal care services to residents living in their own private apartment units. The facility reflects the evolution of residential arrangements for seniors within the system. The hospital first began its effort to capture a larger share of the elderly market in 1985 with the construction of a Section 8 housing complex for low-income elderly on the hospital's campus. Five years later, the hospital added a middle-income elderly independent living housing complex that offered one meal a day and some recreational services. The enriched housing was added five years after that with the construction of a wing to the middle-income independent living complex.

The "mother ship," Health Campus Village's hospital, however, has been struggling financially. Its system has gone through all the chaos of mergers and rapid changes in ownership commonly attributed to publicly traded health care companies. At the time of our visit, negotiations were under way to determine which one of the remaining more dominant health systems in their service area would acquire the hospital system's facilities and whether the residential housing components would be sold separately. The future ownership and direction of the senior services developed by the hospital system and Health Campus Village is unclear.

The independent living complex was originally constructed and managed under contract by a national firm that specializes in the development and construction of senior living facilities. The hospital subsequently chose to manage the development directly. The current executive director of the complex comes to his position from a hospitality background, having previously worked for a national hotel chain. His selection as executive director was a conscious effort to promote the hotel or hospitality attractions of the complex. That emphasis probably contributed to the subsequent complaints of the independent living residents about the enriched housing addition. They did not like being near people who looked so much like nursing home patients. That is not why they had become tenants in the complex. However, as more of their longtime neighbors gravitated to this wing, complaints have given way to visits, shared activities, and a grudging acknowledgment of the advantage it might someday offer them.

The system's senior housing, acute hospital, and nursing homes function independently on a day-to-day basis and have their own boards of directors. However, they are accountable to the overall direction of the system's corporate board, and some back office functions such as purchasing and accounting have been centralized.

The independent living and enriched housing complex were the only private-pay facilities of their type in the area until several years ago. Now, however, new facilities have proliferated in their local service area. A national chain has opened an unlicensed facility specializing in dementia care. Another national chain has constructed a licensed enriched housing facility with a dementia-specific section. In a neighboring more affluent suburban area four or five new assisted living facilities have opened to appeal to the affluent private-pay market. Most of them are owned by the dominant hospital systems in the area. The person involved in setting up Health Campus Village's senior residential services was lured away to assist with this effort.

Health Campus Village also faces some competition from the older licensed adult homes, which have focused on the private-pay market. They have the advantage of being able to care for a somewhat wider range of needs than Health Campus Village's independent living and enriched housing at a lower cost. Yet these adult homes do not have separate apartments. "We don't see these as directly competing with us. Adult children typically do the shopping for individuals that are currently living independently in their own homes, and our units provide an easier and less jarring transition," the director says.

Health Campus Village operates at 98–100% occupancy, and, in part because of its location within a larger system, the director does not anticipate a problem in continuing to operate at that level. It has waiting lists, which the director prefers to describe as a "prospect list." More importantly, almost two thirds of admissions are now internally generated from the independent living complex, hospital, and nursing homes. The system also has a physicians group and an adult day care program, both of which also provide referrals.

Health Campus Village operates with about a 50% turnover in residents each year and an average length of stay of a year and a half. This more rapid turnover and shorter length of stay of residents reflect its location in an integrated delivery system with a much more clearly articulated continuum of care.

Residents typically enter the facility in their mid-eighties, and the average age of residents at the facility is eighty-seven. "Most folks want to stay where they are," the director says. "The children shop ahead of time. They want privacy, security, and to have their parent in a less isolated setting. The first month after relocation, the confusion goes up and there is a lot of sadness, sense of loss, and depression. After three to four months most have made the transition."

FINANCING

Monthly private rates are based on the size of the unit. Residents have the option of hiring private personal care aides and nurses, when they become necessary, but that is arranged privately through the family and typically takes place while awaiting placement. Rates range from $2,414 to $3,008 per month. Each unit has a small kitchen, and the larger units have private porches. Most residents rarely use either, and they seem to be there just to provide the illusion of independent living. Indeed, the stoves in the apartments of those who appear to have some cognitive impairment have been turned off.

The facility, located in a moderate-income suburban area, tries to make its units' prices competitive with other facilities. It fulfills the goal typically established for such new ventures in health systems by generating a small contribution to the operating margin of the system and contributing to the acute hospital admissions. Its profit margin, achieved in part through an efficient floor space design in the apartments and common areas and tight control of staffing costs, is probably less than $50,000 per year.

The flat monthly payments and narrow operating margins discourage admission of prospective residents with complicated care needs. The staff makes a careful assessment of prospects for admission. A nurse participates in the assessment in order to flag medications that may reflect more complicated care needs. The prospective resident must have a minimum degree of self-direction (i.e., must not be cognitively impaired or confused) and be mobile without assistance.

The admission assessment also screens out prospective residents who cannot afford to pay the private rate. Monthly income and assets must be sufficient to assure that the resident can self-pay for at least three years. The facility has never had a resident who was not able to pay. If such a situation occurred, "they wouldn't be put out on the street, but we would aggressively assist them in finding another place," the director said. Private long-term insurance has not been a factor in assuring financial ability to pay. There have been only two individuals in five years of operation for whom private long-term care insurance assisted in paying for their stay.

OPERATIONS

The health system includes an acute hospital and nursing homes. They are separate operations, unlike the linked operations of a continuing care retirement community (CCRC). However, the transition of residents from independent living to enriched housing involves relocation to essentially identical units with shared activities, similar to the way this would work in a CCRC. There is, however, little opportunity for residents in the enriched housing units to age in place. The emphasis of the units is on their role as part of the integrated delivery system rather than encouraging aging in place. Pricing and staffing decisions reflect the difference in the purpose the system is designed to serve.

Responding to the Demands of Assisted Living

A HOME, CHOICE, AND A PLACE TO GROW OLD

The attractively laid out apartments with their own porches and kitchens are no different than the independent living residences in the adjoining complex. Residents choose how to furnish them and enjoy the same privacy as in the independent living complex. There is a set meal schedule, but residents can choose from a menu in the restaurant-like dining room. Some of the activities are combined with those of the independent living residential complex, which is connected by a corridor. Residents can choose activities or just keep to themselves.

Residents have the opportunity to have their voice heard by putting suggestions in a box or expressing their views to a resident council that meets once a month. The director conducts the resident council meetings, which involve information sharing rather than decision making. There are no officers or other trappings of residence self-governance associated with it. "Residents seem reluctant to voice criticisms at this public forum," the activity director said.

The facility follows the regulatory guidelines concerning the rights of residents. Residents can refuse medications, but the facility must notify their physician. "We can't tell the diabetic what they can't do, but we can reason with them," the administrator said. Smoking is not permitted in public areas. If residents have problems leaving stoves on, an addendum to their residency contract is recorded, and the stove is shut off. Residents are free to come and go as they please. One of the residents still drives her automobile. There are no formalized risk contracts and no perceived need for them by the staff. "I have to be careful not to hover. I get concerned about the wanderers," the activities director says.

Residents acknowledge that living in their apartments is different than living in their own homes. "You have to fit in; when you can't, you're out on the street. I am in a group, and I have to comply with the rules, but I can choose what activities I participate in," one resident said. "I am a do-it-yourselfer, and I miss that," one said. "I gave up my car; it is a loss. You have to beg for everything," another said. "There is no place to stay for people that visit," observed another resident.

Yet the facility more than lives up to expectations in meeting residents' most important need. "All I wanted was someone to say, 'I care for you,'" one resident said. "This place is home for me. I am treated as an individual person. . . . My greatest need is for people to be kind and respect me. No arguing. I cried all the way here, but I haven't cried since. You come to a different plateau, and you have to start over."

Most are able to find ways to adapt and find ways to fill some of the losses they felt. "My wife was a musician, and we were in singing groups in churches and at Tanglewood in the summer. I am in the small singing group here. It helps fill the void I feel," said a widower. Others were able to adapt by being more philosophical and relating their experience to earlier ones in their lives. "I spent WW II in the military, and it's a different kind of life like here," said one male resident. The staff is often an important source of strength.

"If there's sadness, they feel your need. They rally around you when you get low, and they seem to know your low points," said a woman who had recently become a resident.

Residents have choices, imperfect and incomplete as they often seemed. "There is regimentation. You have to discipline yourself," one resident explained. "You have three choices for dinner, and they will always make you a sandwich if you don't want any of these. They make stew, not in the way I use to make it. There is too much food, and the meals seem too close together," said another. "You are free to participate or not in the activities, and they are open to ideas. There are movies and popcorn on the weekend and wine hours before dinner, and everyone has a choice of their own physician," said another when asked about the choices they had.

Yet, unlike most of the other private assisted living facilities, there is little aging in place. The health system provides the traditional medical-model continuum of care with its acute and nursing home services. Relocation to the system's other facilities when necessary may, because of geographic proximity, be easier to adjust to than placement in a nursing home or hospital outside the system, but it is not the same as the stability and security offered by a CCRC and does not represent aging in place. The restraints on aging in place appear to be driven by the policies established when the enriched units were developed. They were designed not to compete with other parts of the integrated delivery system. The pricing and, as a consequence, staffing are driven by policies that, in turn, greatly limit the diversity of needs that can be accommodated. The facility, like others faced with similar constraints, is not interested in obtaining waivers to keep residents whose needs exceed the existing level of care and would not change its policies even if the need to obtain waivers were removed. There is a strong financial disincentive to allow aging in place and a strong incentive on the part of the system as a whole to move residents to nursing homes where higher payment can be obtained.

The residents themselves were ambivalent about aging in place and somewhat resigned to being processed along the continuum of care of the system. While they generally expressed a preference for staying, some were not sure whether they would want to stay if they got sicker. "I don't know—we're all living on borrowed time. One lady had a stroke and was found dead in her apartment," one resident said. Resident comments on the facility's discharge policies focused on poor attitudes and failure to comply with the rules rather than on decline in the physical condition of the residents who were discharged. They have less control over their physical condition than their ability to play by the rules, so the prospect of increasing physical dependency was more troubling to think about. "If you are a troublemaker, if you don't go along with the rules, they could discharge you," one said.

Growing dependency in others was hard to accept as well. The activities director reflected on the beginning of blending independent living residents with the enriched housing residents: "When we first started bringing over people from the enriched to the independent living area for activities, we had to deal with a lot of negativism. 'Why are you bringing them over here?' the independent residents would ask. Now some play bingo at both places. The independent living people visit over here."

ASSURING SAFETY AND HIGH STANDARDS OF CARE

Given the admission and discharge policies of Health Campus Village, it is not surprising that the administrator favored retaining licensure with the attendant inspections to the looser arrangements that would only require registration: "If I were a consumer, I would pick a licensed facility." The administrator's frustrations were with the consistency of the surveyors. One surveyor cited the facility for keeping a glass door open because he defined it as a fire door. Previous surveyors ignored this, since it was doubtful that a glass door could serve that function. Yet "It's always nice to have another set of eyes, even if it is a pain sometimes," the administrator noted. Indeed, on a number of occasions, the director and, subsequently, other staff cited external regulations and guidelines shaping what they permit and do not permit their residents to do. The licensure regulations are seen as a resource contributing to the smooth running of the facility rather than as bureaucratic impediments that interfere with responding to the needs of residents.

Yet, in spite of the screening, monitoring, and discharge practices, the staff often feel overstressed in dealing with the increasing fragility of its residents. One staff member observed, "About five of the residents should not be here. Several have incontinence that they can't manage, producing complaints from other residents. One requires total care and should be gone."

As in other facilities, there is friction between the nurse and director, both of whom have plenty of bristle and different assumptions and concerns. The nurse felt that she should have the final say about admissions and discharges and more authority over the personal care aides: "The good ones don't get a lot of respect. They need praise and recognition. Physicians must complete a state-required form for all residents indicating that they can self-medicate, but in many situations this is not the case and we have to arrange to supervise the medications. I distribute the medications, and I am not confident of the aides in most cases to carry this out. I am not happy about the delegation, in some instances, on shifts where I am not present. Some of the aides are not reading the labels, not observing the resident taking the medications. I have nightmares about it."

The personal care aides, in turn, felt forced to fill in where staffing was limited. For example, they fill in as receptionists and activities director on weekends. "We also end up fixing stopped toilets, etc., when we can't get maintenance to come. We end up helping out in the kitchen, adding to our duties." The other theme echoed in our discussion with the personal care aides has to do with respect and recognition. "There needs to be a way to give more recognition and a pat on the back to aides. We had educational programs and in-service training at the hospital, and we should have similar opportunities here," one of the more experienced aides said. "The residents do give us a bonus at Christmas, and the picnics where we bring our families are nice," another observed.

The problems of safety and assuring a high standard of care by Health Campus Village raise important questions. It is unlikely that a surveyor would uncover and address the potentially corrosive tensions between the manager, nurse, and personal care aides regarding the standards of care. The problem may be more structural than interpersonal. Organizing care along a continuum is supposed to assure safety to residents and patients. Individual facilities are only supposed to care for a population within a narrow band of homogenous needs. It is the organizational model that drives the design, pricing, and staffing of Health Campus Village. Yet neither people nor the aging process itself fit neatly into such boxes. The tensions between the nursing director, the manager, and the personal care aides are symptomatic of a rigid structure unable to respond to the diverse and changing needs of residents. Is organizing care along a rigid continuum a greater threat to safety than organizing care to accommodate aging in place? Perhaps more complex adaptive systems work better than the traditional machine-production models.

Shady Oaks

Business Strategy

MARKET NICHE

Shady Oaks is a nonprofit licensed adult home in a suburb. It is a large house in a residential area with beds for more than thirty residents, but it now cares for only half that number. The house is attractive, with a large, beautifully furnished living room and attractively landscaped grounds. It is a real home for its residents. There is little staff turnover. One personal care aide has been there thirty years. The residents and staff feel as if they are all family. There is at least one personal care aide on all shifts. Part-time and per-diem personal care aides are used to give showers, make beds, and just fill in. The staff also includes a nurse consultant who works two days a month, an activities director who works four days a week, and a part-time social worker who doubles as the facility's administrator. A dietician also comes in part-time to assess needs of new residents.

Shady Oaks faces serious occupancy and financial problems. In essence it occupies a niche in the suburban market that no longer exists. It can no longer afford to admit those who cannot afford to pay the private rate, yet it lacks the privacy and amenities now available elsewhere to those who can. Thirty years ago it operated as a health-related facility receiving Medicaid payments. Unable to meet Medicaid standards required of skilled nursing facilities, it reverted to a licensed adult home. It recently merged with another organization. Plans are now under way to build a new eighty-bed adult home close to Shady Oaks and relocate its current residents. The new adult home will also include twenty beds for an assisted living program. However, the new facility will face growing competition and uncertainty about its chances of success.

FINANCING

Until recently, half of the admissions to Shady Oaks were for those who could not afford the private rate. Either they paid on a negotiated sliding-scale basis or the facility accepted the $27 a day or approximately $806 a month from SSI. The other half paid the private rate of $2,058 a month for a single room with a sink. In both cases the flat rate did not go up as the personal care needs of the resident increased.

Shady Oaks no longer accepts any SSI admissions. Yet no one who has run out of money has been discharged. Shady Oaks has never broken even. It cannot raise the private-pay rates without losing more residents. It now carefully reviews the financial resources of prospective residents with the purpose of trying to determine if they can cover the costs for at least a year or two. About 80% of the residents exhaust their financial resources within four years. Shady Oaks is able to continue to operate only because of its sizeable endowment, which subsidizes about half of its budget.

OPERATIONS

Shady Oaks has not reduced its staffing levels to reflect the lower occupancy. This has allowed the facility to meet the growing needs of many of its aging residents. It has let residents die at the home rather than being transferred for that purpose.

The aides and other staff enjoy their work. "What you give, you get in return," one said. There is almost no turnover of staff, and staff members have a comfortable relationship with the facility's administrator. "We are like family," one stated. "We have a good administrator, and we can approach her whenever we want. Her door is always open. She fights for the staff. When we merged, she made sure Shady Oaks remained open and we didn't lose our jobs."

It is a hidden treasure. In spite or perhaps because of all its limitations as a business venture, Shady Oaks embodies much of what advocates, residents, and staff claim to value. Partly as a consequence, it now faces extinction. No margin, no mission.

Responding to the Demands of the Assisted Living

A HOME, CHOICE, AND A PLACE TO GROW OLD

Shady Oaks' vision is what most people would like to see in a "home-like" environment for the frail elderly. However, what limits the attractiveness of Shady Oaks as a "home" is the lack of privacy and private space. The private rooms are eight by twelve feet in size with a sink. The residents can lock their rooms from the inside. Residents must share bathrooms, however. Newer facilities, with which Shady Oaks now competes for private-pay residents, offer full private apartment-like living. Two residents we talked with said they might consider moving if they could get a private bathroom for about the same cost.

It is hard to protect the confidentiality of written information in such a small facility. We saw personal information about residents tacked up on the activity room door for all to see: their diet, doctors, date of birth, and health status. Staff members often speak about residents without realizing others can hear.

The close relationship between staff and residents imposes its own limits on the independence and autonomy of residents. The staff try to persuade residents not to take risks. Those efforts, however, are ad hoc and informal. In rare cases, the facility has asked residents to leave who were unwilling to accept restrictions. For example, there was a man who was confused who wanted to go out every day. It was his habit in his old neighborhood, but the staff was afraid that he would get lost. The family was willing to take that risk, but Shady Oaks was not. The facility told the family he could not stay. In another situation, a woman who was on a medication that is affected by sunlight insisted on sitting in the sun each day. The staff tried to convince her not to, or at least put on sun block. She refused. "I'm retired now, and I want to sit in the sun," she said. They left her alone. Shady Oaks tries to err on the side of safety. It tries to offer alternatives. The close and trusting relationship between staff and residents rarely turns such efforts into a battle of wills. Residents with whom we spoke told us that if the staff told them that something was too risky, they would follow that advice. "I would be stupid not to," said one, surprised at the question. "We try to stay out of their lives as much as possible, but residents go to staff and pull them in," the director said.

Residents do not have a lot of choices. Meals are scheduled at certain times. There is little choice in food. A choice of shower time is offered when the part-time worker comes in to assist with that. While residents can choose their own doctor, they are encouraged to use the physician that regularly visits the facility. There is no resident council. There is a sign asking for suggestions. "The residents know they can come and talk to me at any time," the director says, and the residents we talked with agreed. Some did not like the schedules telling them when they have to eat. They can't sleep as late as they want because they would miss breakfast. "We are dependent on outsiders," one said.

The residents are mostly homebound. "We have tried to take them out. Recently we were successful in getting them out to a kindergarten graduation one block away with children who are part of the intergenerational project they are involved in. The children invited them to their graduation, and the residents did not want to disappoint the children," the director said. The facility does try to bring the community to the residents. A local women's organization works on activities, and the Rotary Club conducts bingo games. The facility's activity program includes fitness every morning, bingo, entertainment, a beauty parlor with free manicuring, horticulture therapy, planting, a choral group, and film videos.

The staff goes the extra mile to do whatever is necessary to allow residents to age in place. A widow lived in the facility for more than sixteen years. She was deteriorating, and state surveyors were concerned.

The staff dressed her and helped her when state inspectors were around. They wanted her to stay. Finally, the facility reached the limits of its ability to care for her, and she was transferred to a nursing home. "As people get sicker, it affects the whole community. It takes away from other people's care," the director said. "I don't want to be around a lot of very sick people, but don't want to ask anyone to leave," one resident said.

ASSURING SAFETY AND HIGH STANDARDS OF CARE

The director had a low opinion of the proposal to offer the option of merely registering homes: "Allowing only registration is crazy. I can hide the things I do and I'm licensed! There must be minimum standards." Even though home health agencies are licensed, she has no faith in the home care agencies' ability to oversee care. "The supervisors are never around," she said.

A nurse consultant, with much experience working in long-term care settings, comes in two days a month to check on the residents. She reviews the charts before the doctor comes in. One physician serves as the doctor for most of the residents. She checks the residents once a month. The nurse consultant makes note of problems and trains the personal care aides to observe issues and document them in nurses' notes. She uses the same record-keeping model she used with nursing homes. While she gives informal counseling to the staff, she has no authority to make the staff do anything. She has a good working relationship with all of them and is pleased with the care they provide.

None of the residents can self-medicate, although this is one of the requirements for admission and retention in an adult home. Aides watch the residents take the medication and document it. The nurse consultant oversees the process. While she has a good working relationship with the doctor who visits regularly, she has a hard time getting through on the phone to some of the residents' other physicians.

The aides are knowledgeable caregivers. They are careful to observe residents, and when they see problems, they call the doctor directly. If, for example, a resident suddenly becomes incontinent, they consult with both the doctor and the director to see if any change in medication might be causing it. One of the simple rules essential for high-quality care proposed by the IOM report summarized in the last chapter is the importance of the free flow of information and the cooperation between caregivers. Of all the facilities discussed in this chapter, this one best exemplifies that rule.

Assessing the Long-Term Impact of Private-Market Assisted Living

Does the growth of private-market assisted living merely reflect the growing economic disparities in care for the frail elderly, or does it offer a new model with the potential for transforming care for all? The five private-pay assisted living facilities surveyed in this chapter support both hypotheses.

Developers try to package their projects to give the appearance of high-status affluence. Seniors and their adult children associate nursing homes with the shame and stigma of the almshouse. Developers know that to sell their product they must avoid that image. They pay a premium to build at prestige addresses and adorn their entranceways with opulent-looking glass chandeliers. Community relations directors and the marketing staff work hard to portray the services they provide in a positive way. They liken their facilities to exclusive resort hotels with extra services. Through the glossy pictures in their brochures, they associate their facilities with the time-tested sales appeal of high social status and eternal youth. Yet success in creating this illusion generates a backlash. Some residents feel they have been tricked, that the number of residents with cognitive impairments and problems with ambulation and incontinence make their new residence a nursing home and not the lively social resort promised in the brochures. Others, associating this level of disability with indigence, suspect that some of their new companions are public charges whom they are subsidizing.

Yet there are not enough individuals who can afford high-cost facilities, and too many developers are trying to capture that end of the market. They can't count on sustained growth in demand for their product. They face boom and bust cycles and fierce competition. Harbor View, an older for-profit adult home, is planning a lavish new development complete with a multistoried atrium and an Olympic swimming pool to meet its new competition. Others, such as Shady Oaks, the small suburban adult home, seem to offer so much in the way of personalized care and a homelike environment, but these fall by the wayside, unable to compete with the privacy and amenities newer facilities can offer. The typical residents in the private assisted living facilities are not the affluent members of a leisure class elite as sometimes implied in assisted living brochures. They are not the Rose Kennedys or the Ronald Reagans. For the most part, they are average people with average pensions and savings. They and their children wince at the costs, and most live in fear of what will happen when the money runs out. They share the same worries and concerns of those who cannot afford private-market assisted living in the first place.

Indeed, the trappings of high-end facilities don't seem very central to their lives as residents. Most rarely use the porches, rockers, kitchenettes, and game rooms, which seem more like stage props. Residents say their relationships with the staff who provide their direct care is by far the most important thing. It was the most frequently mentioned source of satisfaction, and losing their current caregivers was cited as a possible reason they might choose to leave. The caregivers' empathy and the trust that residents have in them is what matters most to the residents of these facilities. The better caregivers understand this and say they want to give the same care they would like to receive when their turn comes. Yet, as one of the aides in Harbor View ironically observed, when their turn comes, they will only be able to afford a space in the parking lot. The economic disparity between residents and caregivers inevitably fosters resentment and strains the relationship that is so important to residents. Perhaps it argues for a common self-interest in assuring something closer to universal access to a single standard of care.

In any event, the growth of private-market assisted living has helped set in motion many changes in the organization of services for the frail elderly. Traditional health care providers are struggling with the impact of these changes. Some hospital systems, such as the one that created Health Campus Village, have tried to use their senior housing to capture a larger share of the acute hospital market and possibly an expanding share of the elderly managed care market. The hospital and nursing home components of such operations face growing financial pressures. A recent examination of the audited financial statements of New York City's nonspecialty hospitals for 1997–1999 revealed that eleven of the city's thirty-six voluntary hospitals face financial problems serious enough to threaten their survival (United Hospital Fund 2001). Nursing homes located in more affluent suburban areas across the country, which have long depended on a proportion of private-pay patients, now face declining occupancies and operating margins. Private-pay assisted living is contributing to a death spiral from which many hospitals, nursing homes, and integrated delivery systems are now struggling to extricate themselves. The market is working, and the landscape of care is changing.

The next chapter examines facilities that offer assisted living for the majority of people who cannot afford to pay the private-market rates for their care. These facilities also have a role to play in determining whether the economic disparities in elderly care will continue and grow or whether we will develop a converging common vision of equitable care for all.

6
Publicly Supported Assisted Living

> Over the hill to the poorhouse I'm trudgin' my weary way—
> I, am woman of seventy, and only a trifle gray—
> I, who am smart an' chipper, for all the years I've told,
> As many another woman that's only half as old.
> Over the hill to the poorhouse—I can't quite make it clear!
> Over the hill to the poorhouse—it seems so horrid queer!
> Many a step I've taken a-toilin' to and fro,
> But this is a sort of journey I never thought to go.
> What is the use of heapin' on me a pauper's shame?
> Am I lazy or crazy? Am I blind or lame?
> —Will Carelton, "Over the Hill to the Poorhouse"

"Over the Hill to the Poorhouse," familiar lines to all at the beginning of the twentieth century, captures the fear and shame of institutionalization in old age, still present at the beginning of the twenty-first century. What do we owe to the elderly? Is poverty in old age a crime that should be punished by imprisonment? Do individuals in a community have value beyond what they can command in the market? What kind of community do we have if they don't? The Social Security legislation of the 1930s and the Medicare legislation of the 1960s mandated basic income security for the elderly and held that they and their families should be spared impoverishment by medical expenses in old age. Yet it has proven to be a difficult promise to honor. The nursing home, the dominant component of our long-term care system, still receives most of its income from public medical assistance (Medicaid). It inherited the role of the poorhouse and has yet to shake off that shadow of the past. All but the most affluent of private-pay assisted living facility residents will take the journey over the hill to the poorhouse if they live long enough.

The specter of the almshouse remains as a result of deliberate public policy decisions. Public policies have pushed to control cost by making publicly supported care an unattractive choice of last resort. Nursing homes have become medicalized settings, restricted to the most seriously incapacitated. Care for the indigent frail elderly has shifted to less costly settings such as adult homes or boarding homes and low-income housing where services have been added. While these facilities and programs that care for the indigent elderly meet the broad definition of assisted living, few would be confused with those serving the private market in terms of their physical amenities. Unlike hospitals, nursing homes' and medical practices' care for private-pay and publicly supported residents takes place in an almost completely separate set of facilities.

The facilities that provide assisted living care for the indigent elderly in New York State are similar to those elsewhere in the nation. They include adult homes, boarding homes, and low-income housing programs that care for increasingly frail elderly residents. Some states have obtained Medicaid waivers that allow payment for the care of nursing home–eligible patients in home- and community-based settings. New York, in a minor variation on this approach, created assisted living programs (ALPs). New York State certifies a small number of existing enriched housing programs and adult homes that work with licensed home health agencies to provide a nursing home level of care as ALPs. The New York State Medicaid program provides partial nursing home payments to these ALPs for patients who need care similar to that provided in a nursing home. Since licensure is a condition for public payment to any type of assisted living facility, the facilities receiving these payments cannot elude licensure as some exclusively private-pay facilities in New York have done.

In terms of their missions, these facilities share much in common with those serving the private-pay market. Most of the operators of these facilities feel they are part of the same movement, trying to give lower-income people the same choices and the homelike settings now being marketed to those who can afford to pay privately. This chapter assesses the ability of five different public-pay facilities to provide assisted living services. Three urban facilities, one suburban, and one exurban facility will be described. Like their five private counterparts described in the previous chapter, some are more like private housing and some more closely resemble nursing homes. The facilities described in this chapter are identified by the following pseudonyms:

1. Senior Apartments: A public-pay, nonprofit licensed enriched housing program in New York City that is integrated into a long-term care delivery system.
2. Assisted Living Program Housing: A public-pay, nonprofit, licensed enriched housing assisted living program operating in an upstate urban setting.
3. City Towers Home: A public-pay, proprietary-owner-operated licensed adult home assisted living program in New York City.
4. Green Acres Apartments: A public-pay, nonprofit licensed enriched housing program located in the suburbs of New York City.
5. Farm Home: A public-pay, proprietary-owner-operated licensed adult home serving psychiatric and elderly residents in a small-town upstate setting.

Altogether, these five facilities encompass most of the diversity in publicly supported assisted living as it currently exists in the United States.

Senior Apartments

Business Strategy

MARKET NICHE

Senior Apartments is an enriched housing program. It is part of a large nursing home and hospital complex in New York City. The program has twenty apartments scattered throughout a large apartment complex for fully independent seniors. These are studio and one-bedroom apartments. While they are currently full, the number of vacancies has fluctuated over the last few years. If an apartment is not occupied quickly, it may revert to independent living housing. The program is promoted to professional social workers. Most of the referrals come either from the integrated delivery system itself or from a variety of other agencies, shelters, and subacute units in the area. The program conducts extensive screening of applicants with a social worker and a psychiatrist and limits admissions to cognitively unimpaired persons who need housing.

FINANCING

Senior Apartments does not admit any private-pay residents. It admits only those who are eligible for Supplemental Security Income (SSI). It receives $799 a month for each resident. The program loses $40,000 a year when fully occupied. The loss was higher until the food service was changed. The program now gets all of its food from the nursing home; the food includes prepared dinners and groceries for breakfast and lunch, which are made by the residents. The residents were unhappy about the change and complained about the lower quality of food. The director believes that the costs of the program cannot be cut any more and that it will continue to operate at a deficit even though the nursing home now absorbs all of the food costs.

OPERATIONS

Senior Apartments uses the licensed home care agency that is part of the hospital and nursing home complex. The agency employs three aides to do the housekeeping and shopping and serve the food. If residents need more than these services (six hours a week of aide time, one meal a day), they can receive additional home care on a fee-for-service basis though the Medicaid program.

The program's connection with the nursing home allows for the use of the nursing home's adult day care and therapy services. The program embraces the basic medical continuum-of-care model. Medical professionals make the decisions about care. If a resident is getting sicker or refuses to comply with the rules, the resident is quickly transferred to the nursing home. However, staff did give examples of their working to keep a resident, usually after the resident's family insisted.

If a resident has a medical problem between 9:00 A.M. and 5:00 P.M., there are many professionals ready to help him; if a medical problem occurs after hours, a resident must push the call button, which is answered by the security guard in the lobby. The guard calls 911, and the resident is taken to the hospital to be checked out. In the daytime Senior Apartments functions like a health facility and at night like a private apartment complex. The residents would prefer on-site care to the nighttime emergency arrangement.

The ambiguity of the boundaries between independent housing and the care program in this particular facility creates conflicts. Legally the tenant rights of the resident take precedence over the contract with the enriched housing program. For example, if a resident is no longer able to continue to participate in the program, he can continue to stay in the apartment as a tenant. Assisted living facilities and programs typically insist on contracts with residents that take precedence over any presumed rights as tenants. The decision regarding when the individual can no longer be cared for in the facility is left to the sole discretion of the facility. In this respect, residents in Senior Apartments have greater rights than the residents of any of the private facilities described in the previous chapter. Private assisted living facility contracts usually require only thirty days' notice to residents but also allow for immediate discharge or eviction when the facility determines that continued residence represents an immediate threat to the life of the individual or other residents.

Responding to the Demands of Assisted Living

PROVIDING A HOME, CHOICE, AND A PLACE TO GROW OLD

This "boutique" program is one of only a few in which low-income elderly residents enjoy the private apartment living that is the standard among facilities catering to the private market. The residents were generally pleased with their "homes." One man was delighted; he did not have a home when he moved there and was glad just to have a roof over his head. One of the women residents felt relieved to be there. She liked the sense of community in the apartment complex. Most residents' complaints centered on food. They did not like to have dinner at one specific time. Most knew whom to complain to but felt it did not make any difference. All felt that there was not enough staff. Only one person serves dinner, and the food gets cold. The residents like the staff and feel that the staff know the residents well. But if an emergency arises and a resident needs to be taken to a doctor, others will not get their apartments cleaned.

Residents join activities with clients of the geriatric outreach program for members of the surrounding community. They can participate in any of the activities and can also go next door to the nursing home for any of the activities there. In addition, the Senior Apartments residents have their own separate activities, which include seeing movies, visiting museums, taking boat rides, and parties. Most have families who visit frequently. Some of the residents are active in neighborhood churches and synagogues.

Privacy is protected in that residents live alone in apartments. "We have morning rounds every day where aides knock on doors and wait to hear that all are OK," said one of the personal care aides. Residents can keep their doors locked, and all charts are kept locked in the Senior Apartments office.

While the dinner menu is limited, residents are given an extensive list of foods to choose from for groceries and a menu to fill out for dinner. They also receive $28 in food stamps that they can use for purchases of their own choosing. They have all the autonomy and freedom that any other apartment dweller has. They are not forced to participate in activities, and visitors can come at any time. There is no resident council, but residents meet weekly as a group to discuss issues.

As apartment dwellers, residents can take many risks. "We try to find out why a resident is taking risks at our team meeting. We try to convince the resident not to take risks. If a resident chooses to do unsafe things, we speak to them and their physician," the director said.

Senior Apartments takes a conservative approach to aging in place and risks. Prospective residents are carefully screened, weeding out those who cannot physically care for themselves or who are cognitively impaired. Most of the residents agree with this approach. "I wouldn't want to live with others who were cognitively impaired or a hazard to the community," said one resident. Residents can refuse services, but some control is imposed through the standing orders observed by the staff in their daily routine. For example, one woman fell off her bed reaching for something; a staff member who happened to be in her room insisted on calling the nurse even though the resident said she felt fine. The nurse in turn insisted on sending the resident to the hospital even though she did not want to go. If the resident had fallen out of bed at night with no staff around, she would simply have gone back to bed. The program is careful about assuming risks. For example, one resident was becoming demented. She also wandered. Senior Apartments wanted to place her elsewhere. Her son objected. Senior Apartments worked to find her an "appropriate" placement. Sometimes a resident's family is asked to supply caregiving if needed in order to keep the resident in the program.

ASSURING SAFETY AND HIGH STANDARDS OF CARE

"There needs to be regulations; however there needs to be reasonable discussion when surveys are taking place," the administrator of the program said. For example, Senior Apartments gets no money for nursing supervisors, yet the state sets standards related to medication under nurse supervision. The primary way Senior Apartments assures quality of care is by careful professional screening of applicants and ongoing monitoring of residents. The program tries to attract people who have difficulty living alone or who are living in an unsafe situation but are still very much cognitively intact. Most residents can accomplish basic tasks of daily living (bathing, dressing, eating, etc.). What they need is limited supervision, someone checking on their eating, cleanliness, and so forth. Senior Apartments regularly reviews the individual care plans of residents. Much of that responsibility falls to the nurse, who works about sixteen hours a week overseeing the care of residents. She sees her role as following up on clients who are using medications after hospitalization or who need frequent blood sugar or blood pressure tests. She also meets once a month with all residents to discuss health issues. Medications are put into a weekly medical set for the residents. She checks to make sure that they are not running out of their prescription; if they are, she reorders. She does not give out medication and does not check on whether medication is actually taken.

Assisted Living Program Housing

Business Strategy

MARKET NICHE

Assisted Living Program Housing is a licensed enriched housing ALP. The agency that operates the ALP manages other enriched housing sites in apartment complexes owned by this Upstate New York housing authority. They make rent payments for the residents in the units for which they are responsible. The ALP is part of an enriched housing site developed by the conversion and renovation of a solidly constructed building. The agency was able to get a waiver from the Department of Housing and Urban Development, which requires a mix of enriched and independent housing units, to convert what was originally designed as fifteen enriched housing units and fifteen independent living units to all enriched housing. Then, two years ago, an ALP was approved for fifteen of the facility's residents.

Assisted Living Program Housing is located in a high-crime inner-city area. Many of the houses in the neighborhood are in poor repair. According to the director, drug activity and occasional shootings take place in the general proximity of this attractively renovated building. Visitors sometimes call and ask fearfully, "Where can I park my car?"

Reflecting on this program's market niche, the director says, "Our competition is from the PACE programs that get all-inclusive capitated rates of $4,000 per month or more and the residents have to go to day care. As far as enriched housing and enriched housing ALPs for SSI recipients in this area, we are it. The adult homes are not our competition, since access for SSI recipients to the decent ones in this area is very limited. The geographic location is a problem for some prospective residents and their families. They ask why couldn't you be in another part of the city? Well, the real estate is affordable here for a program like this."

Many of the program's referrals are generated from the other enriched housing sites operated by the same agency. Other applicants are referred from the hospitals, home care agencies, and the city's adult protective services. The director says, "The hospital discharge planners and agency people know about us. We don't advertise because we don't have the need or the budget. Residents in the enriched housing programs have first priority into the ALP. We currently have four individuals on a waiting list; we get three to four vacancies per year, but it is unpredictable. Some residents have lived with us for more than ten years. It is also a very heterogenous group; we have residents from the mid-fifties through the late nineties. Most don't have a lot of family, and those that do have problems with them."

FINANCING

The $27 a day for those on SSI does not cover the costs, which are $43 a day. The facility leases units for residents from the city housing authority and pays their rent in a lump sum. The rent for SSI recipients is $170 a month, 30% of their SSI. The income from an SSI recipient for enriched housing is $776 per month ($170 for rent, $606 to cover the cost of the program). SSI also provides about $40 per month for personal incidentals. A private-pay enriched housing resident at the facility with a monthly income of about $1,000 would pay $300 for rent and $700 to cover the cost of the program, so the facility "makes" a little more on these residents, but at the time of our interviews, the facility had only one private-pay resident. A voluntary agency charitable donation subsidizes the resulting deficit of the program at about $175,000 per year. "Our argument is that we are saving the taxpayers the greater cost of nursing home placement by delaying such placements," the director says. For the ALP-eligible residents, the numbers are much better. ALP patients receive 60% of the Medicaid nursing home rate plus the SSI payment. These combined payments range from $72 to $82 a day.

OPERATIONS

Nevertheless, the program strains to provide the services that the ALP residents need within its budget. The staff often gets involved in looking for loopholes that can make a large difference in the costs that the facility incurs for residents. For example, a resident with a stage three pressure ulcer on her heel required a visit from the home health agency to change the dressing at a cost of $80 per day, which had to be absorbed by the program. Transporting the resident to a wound clinic at a local hospital, however, eliminated this cost, because the clinic bills Medicare directly for its services. After a hospitalization, the program has to pay for the follow-up care by a home health agency. However, if the residents are sent to a nursing home for a short-term rehabilitation stay, Medicare pays the costs. Costs are also shaved by aides' working only thirty hours a week on four shifts for $7.14 an hour. The pay, the open-ended nature of the job, and the demands sometimes placed upon the staff by residents create friction between the aides, their supervisors, and the residents. There is frequent turnover of aides. However, this was the only sour note. The ALP apartments are attractive and spacious. The building is well maintained. There is a rich and diverse activities program, an active resident council, good monitoring of the needs of residents, and a friendly, homelike atmosphere.

Responding to the Demands of Assisted Living

PROVIDING A HOME, CHOICE, AND A PLACE TO GROW OLD

The spacious high-ceiling apartments the low-income residents of Assisted Living Program Housing occupy would be the envy of most Manhattan apartment dwellers. They are real homes, private apartments, which are furnished often in loving detail by the residents. Assisted Living Program Housing compares favorably to private-market operations in terms of floor space and staffing ratios. Although the amenities of food preparation and physical surroundings may be less than ideal, the care is essentially the same as that offered in private-pay assisted living facilities.

The activities director said, "Art therapy is a difficult idea for these people who have never viewed themselves as artistic or creative. You have to break through barriers. Poetry helps, and a variety of games. Games that are especially useful are ones with surprise that create laughter—such as balloon tennis with flyswatters and tabletop bowling. The women were more reluctant participants at first. The games involve lots of applause and laughter. Activities can involve as many as half the residents if food is available. There is also a men's and a women's group; Sunday afternoon there is a movie with popcorn and soda. Outings include lunch out once a month, participation with a fifth-grade class, and visits to art galleries, picnics, and the zoo."

What makes Assisted Living Program Housing distinctive from all the other private and public facilities we visited, however, is the strong sense of ownership and control felt by its residents. The tenants' council is the only one we encountered that is operated by tenants with their own elected officers. Fifteen residents actively participate. They focus on maintenance, food, and decisions related to the decoration of the common areas. They keep minutes.

Part of this sense of ownership is explained by the history of the housing complex and the distinctive culture that evolved. It began as independent housing and later added enriched housing. Additional services responded to the aging in place of residents in much the way that some naturally occurring retirement communities (NORCs) have adapted to similar aging of their residents. Because of this evolution, the tenants have long been accustomed to running things. The "old guard" did not welcome the transition to an ALP. It was not so much that some of the newer residents were frailer and sicker but that the old guard felt it was beginning to lose control of the after-hours life of the place where they use to have free rein, with night card games and drinking. "The building would rock and roll" the director said. Now there is staff on the premises twenty-four hours a day. There was a struggle over who was in charge. Residents complained that the staff was ordering them around. That struggle of wills created, as described by the staff, "a resident-empowered institutional culture." The staff, or at least the administrators, took pride in the creation of this distinctive culture. Yet in a very real sense, the residents trained the staff to conform to their expectations rather than vice versa. There is an object lesson in this. Perhaps assisted living that evolves like NORCs is more likely to resist externally designed institutional cultures and permit the persistence of resident-centered control.

For whatever reason, the facility has bent to the demands of its residents. "We promote independence and empowerment," the administrator said. "The only controls are related to state and county regulations governing smoking and life safety. These are adults, and we're not running a kids program. We are dealing with a population that have been risk takers all of their lives. They have had their share of heavy drinking and gambling. Some are tinkerers that create safety hazards in the apartments that upset the fire safety inspectors. There is a legally blind ninety-year-old lady that has an antique lamp that she uses to hang clothes in her apartment. She was cited for a violation by the fire inspector. The next time he came for an inspection, she took out a scissors and clipped off the plug from the cord. 'There! It's a coat hanger now and not a lamp!'"

Residents are free to have guests but are encouraged to inform staff when they do. "An aide walked into an apartment on the third floor of one of our female residents and found a naked man in bed," the director related. "The resident appeared from the bathroom. We like residents to let us know about visitors to avoid such embarrassments." One resident in his eighties was involved in his younger years on the periphery of organized crime. He is sometimes out with his old gambling buddies until early morning. "About half the residents have intact families and regular visitors. For the rest, we are their family," the director said.

Independent apartments imply the assumption of risk-taking by residents. Physicians are notified if medical regimens or dietary restrictions of residents are violated, but nothing like a formalized risk contract exists or is under consideration. The director says, "There is a woman resident who used to work as a waitress in a bar and is used to staying up late and taking her sleeping pill at 1:30 A.M. We arrange for this. The lack of involved family members limits the need for such negotiations. Most of the residents either have no family in the area or are estranged from them. Indeed, state regulations protect the ability of residents to refuse medications and, in the process, protect the facility against the bad outcomes that might result."

As they become more dependent, residents can progress from independent living to enriched housing to the ALP within units operated by the agency. However, the separate apartment units and the freedom of residents to come and go as they please limit the nature of the population that can effectively age in place in this setting. It is not an appropriate site for Alzheimer's patients. It is ideal for medically complex, cognitively intact self-ambulating residents who have a fierce desire to maintain their independence.

"There are a some residents that have exceeded our ability to care for them and the tolerance of the other residence. There was a resident with dementia who would stay in her room. She became very anxious, and we became concerned about safety. We were afraid she would not have been self-directing in event of a fire. We had reached the limits with a younger individual with MS. We had to do two-person transfers. She was hospitalized as a result of her rapidly worsening condition, and we didn't have to force the issue. We also have a schizophrenic, obsessive-compulsive person that we have been struggling with. It takes a lot of time to get him to the doctor. He disrupts the dinner seating arrangements. He can be aggravating to staff and other residents. We are trying to work on this case. Yet he's an example of a case that would be impossible to manage without his own private apartment where he can exert control. There was also the resident who smashed another resident over the head with a chair. We evicted him. This one was clear; it exceeded the boundary of what was acceptable/defensible in terms of the safety of the residents. Incontinence is not a problem, if at least partially self-managing. One resident began placing feces in candy dishes, and this required placement elsewhere. It wasn't the incontinence; it was the psychotic behavior that made this necessary."

ASSURING SAFETY AND HIGH STANDARDS OF CARE

The program is comfortable working with the rules imposed externally by the housing authority, the life safety code, and state enriched housing and ALP regulations. Indeed, in a very real sense, the staff views regulation as an ally, imposing limits on the absolute autonomy of residents without undermining their philosophy of assuring residents the most independence possible. Staff members of this facility questioned whether for-profit facilities could make the right choices about the care, admission, and retention of residents if such external controls were eliminated. "No, I don't like it. I don't like to set people up for failure. It shouldn't be up to the facility," the nursing director said. "Other motives enter in. The waiver arrangement makes sense. You need to assure a minimum standard. People for whom this would work have to be cognitively intact and have a real drive to remain independent. This is a very diverse industry, and if the prime motivation is the bottom line or return to stockholders, I would not want to simply leave it up to the facility.

"The mix is good. They look after each other. The crew goes shopping. It is doubtful that the disabled would venture out without the others. One resident who is legally blind got on the wrong bus and got lost, which worried us and all the other residents, but he eventually got back."

The registered nurse dispenses medications. Delegating this task to aides did not work, and the administrator and nursing director are dubious about its ability to work in other settings. The additional ALP Medicaid dollars support the service for both the ALP and enriched housing residents. The resident council serves as another important form of quality assurance in this setting.

Morale and recruitment of personal care aides, however, is a major weak link in this program. There is ongoing friction between the aides, their supervisors, and the residents. The low pay, the degree of resident control, and the expanding open-endedness of their work create a volatile situation. "People here put on airs. They don't need as much care as they think," one personal care aide said. Part of the problem is the personalities of the residents. "This is an abrupt, very demanding group. Some can be very cruel to aides," the nursing director said. The strong sense of control the residents have is at the expense of the aides. Addressing one problem impinges on addressing another.

City Towers Home

Business Strategy

MARKET NICHE

City Towers Home is a licensed for-profit adult home with more than two hundred beds. The interior of the building is well maintained and attractive. The exterior has a bleak, institutional appearance and lacks any landscaping that would soften the urban surroundings. Half the beds provide care for the traditional adult home residents and half for those who are eligible for the Medicaid ALP. The ALP has been in existence for about five years and took only six months to reach full capacity. Most rooms are double with a shared bathroom. The major competitors are other ALPs and nursing homes in the city. City Towers Home gets referrals from hospitals and geriatric-related social service agencies, but it does not accept psychiatric patients. The director of development, as the community relations person is referred to, insists that she does not market. She "educates people about what assisted living is and what our facility has to offer."

While the home has been able to maintain full occupancy, the administrators would prefer more private-pay residents. The proportion of private-pay residents has dropped from about 40% to 30%. The opening of attractive private assisted living facilities that offer a greater degree of privacy has reduced the facility's private-pay admissions. The ALP payments, however, have helped the financial situation. A resident can go from the adult home to the ALP in this facility without changing rooms or even beds. The resident who transfers to the ALP simply gets more nursing care.

FINANCING

The ALP Medicaid payments keep this facility, which combines a minority of private-pay residents with public-pay ones, afloat. If a resident comes in paying privately and spends down, the facility helps the resident apply for public funding and does not discharge the resident. The facility has no formal documentation or procedures to determine financial eligibility. The staff simply ask questions to determine if applicants are eligible for SSI. They tell their private rate to the family. If the family convinces them they do not have enough to pay the private rate, they will discuss a sliding scale. Many families supplement the SSI rate. In essence, their private rates are limited by what their private-pay residents can afford and by the market rates of comparable facilities in the area. Overall, the facility's costs for the ALP residents are about $104 per day. The private and ALP Medicaid payments make up the difference between that cost and the much lower SSI payments for the facility's adult home residents.

OPERATIONS

ALP residents and adult home residents are interspersed and hard to distinguish. In essence, the ALP provides a safety-valve subsidy, assuring adequate support for an adult home population that has growing personal care and health-related needs with the help of federal Medicaid matching funds rather than having the state absorb the full cost through an expansion of the state supplement for SSI recipients. In the process, City Towers Home has achieved a tenuous balance. It is the only facility we visited that has been successful in maintaining a significant mix of private-pay and public-pay residents. The operator says, "You don't need Atlantic City–type lavish common areas to provide good care. The key is maintaining solid relationships with residents and meeting with them constantly. Home care is only good if you have a dedicated and involved family that can check in on things regularly. An adult home provides a similar environment for home care."

Responding to the Demands of Assisted Living
PROVIDING A HOME, CHOICE, AND A PLACE TO GROW OLD

Most rooms are double with a shared bathroom. The facility has an attractive dining area and activity space on the first floor. There are institutional sitting areas on each of five floors—plastic chairs along walls in front of a TV set. The light is good and the overall ambiance is adequate, but the exterior stark.

Most of the residents had a hard time explaining how they had come to this facility. Most did not participate in the decision. In some cases the decision was made by adult protective services. In other cases, the hospital social work staff made the arrangements. City Towers Home takes people who do not choose to come. When we spoke with residents, we found that they are told it will be temporary, and then they stay. One said, "I was at a hospital. I was told that I couldn't live alone and would be at the facility only for a short time. It has now been four years." Another said, "I don't know. I was living in a hotel. The administrator came and got me after the doctor talked me into it. I asked the administrator where he was taking me." In other cases the resident's daughter visited the facility and decided. Most of the residents had no idea what to expect. "I was overwhelmed by the size and the people," one said.

The privacy of having one's own home is lacking. Roommates of adult home residents who become ALP residents complain that too many staff come into their rooms. Supervisors explain to staff that they need to knock before entering rooms. Sometimes residents change their rooms so they can have a non-ALP roommate and a modicum of privacy. The residents we spoke with missed such things as going to the refrigerator at night for a snack, going out after dark, the privacy of a private bathroom, and closet space. "I had to just leave so many of my belongings," one resident said.

Like other facilities we visited, City Towers Home tries to dissuade residents from risky behavior. It is an informal process; there are no formal risk contracts. The staff finds ways to stop people who insist on risky behavior. Sometimes a staff member is sent with someone who wants to go out. The facility has paid residents five dollars to accompany other residents in a car service to keep an eye on them when they go for doctors' appointments. The facility also calls families and gets them involved. Most of the residents say they would not do anything that the staff thought was unsafe.

The resident council meets once a month. It provides an opportunity for residents' complaints to be heard. In order to get people to attend the resident council, the facility turns off the TV and holds meetings right before lunch outside the dining room.

The activities director tries to provide choices for the residents. There are barbecues, a daily exercise program, and games such as Trivial Pursuit, bingo, bowling, and cards. The staff has started organizing outings. The activities program also provides arts and crafts, a cooking class, women's and men's clubs, and gardening activities.

Residents maintain some of the autonomy and choice they would have in their own home. They are offered substitutes for food that they do not like. While they are assigned a table in the dining hall, they can request to be reassigned. They can choose an outside physician or home health agency for care, but few do. Some couples have asked to room together and have been accommodated. One roommate complained that her roommate had a man come in during the night. The administrator suggested that he take her to his room. The facility does not allow overnight guests and confiscates alcohol.

Residents have gotten much frailer at this facility in recent years, and walkers and canes are more in evidence in the hallways. The ALP has helped to allow residents to age in place. About 80% of the ALP residents are former adult home residents of the facility who have aged in place. If a resident needs more care than the ALP can provide, he or she will be transferred to a nursing home, where many die within a few months. City Towers Home does not want to look like a nursing home and will not keep people who require wheelchairs. The facility follows a social rather than a medical model. The residents we spoke with say they want to stay if they can be cared for. It is the "undesirables" who should be discharged. Those who fight, use bad language, break the rules, and create trouble will be kicked out.

ASSURING SAFETY AND HIGH STANDARDS OF CARE

The administrator said that he would like to see unlicensed facilities remain unlicensed. Other facilities becoming licensed means more competition for him. He felt that the ALP should remain as it is. However, he felt that facilities sometimes unfairly receive deficiencies when the home health agency is really at fault.

The facility has a full-time nurse who serves as the director of patient care services. Before coming to this facility, she had worked as a nurse in home care agencies, hospitals, and nursing homes for more than ten years. The major staff challenge she sees is getting staff to understand the ALP residents, most of whom have dementia. "Even though they are here," she said, "they are not in prison. We can't set all the rules." The ALP residents have twice as many staff as the adult home residents. The aides say they love to work with the residents. They feel needed. The facility does not seem to have problems recruiting and keeping staff. In addition to the nurse who serves as director of patient care, the facility also has two physicians; one visits three times a week and the other once a week. There are two psychiatrists and a psychotherapist who help supervise the care.

Medication administration, however, gives the impression of a grim institutional ritual in this setting. Residents line up at mealtimes to get their medication from a trained medication aide. Each patient's medication has a number of paper clips that indicates how often the resident should take the medication. The aide puts the pills in a cup and pours them into the resident's hand. The resident keeps moving down the line to another aide who hands them water. If a resident does not arrive to get the medication, the speaker blares out his name to come down for his medication. The facility lacks some of the safety and protections of a nursing home and some of the graciousness and amenities of a private-pay assisted living facility.

Green Acres Apartments

Business Strategy

MARKET NICHE

A suburban county nonprofit community services agency operates Green Acres Apartments. It consists of two apartments that provide enriched housing for eight frail elderly persons. Each has a private bedroom. The apartments are part of an attractively landscaped cooperative housing development that includes two hundred to three hundred apartments in two-story buildings. Established more than fifty years ago, the community services agency now provides mental health clinics, home health care, and residential care for the developmentally disabled. Its total annual operating expenses are close to $20 million; the two apartments represent only a small component of its operations. The first-floor apartment houses the most physically frail residents and the common dining area for the residents of both apartments. This enriched housing operation has existed with little administrative attention. Its size makes it almost invisible within the larger residential housing program for the developmentally disabled.

There is no effort to market the program; not even a brochure is available. The program has remained fully occupied for a long time, but vacancies are unpredictable. As a result, it sometimes takes several months to find an appropriate replacement. More than half the residents have a history of treatment for mental illness. The large proportion of residents with a history of mental health treatment reflects the informal referral pattern from the agency's large mental health outpatient presence in the community. The agency has chosen to maintain a low profile for its apartments for the developmentally disabled, including Green Acres, which may be an attempt to avoid fueling the fears of residential neighbors. It represents an anomaly. The facility provides a homelike residential setting to a frail elderly SSI population in a residential setting that is neither age- nor income-segregated.

FINANCIALS

The program has existed on its present scale for twenty years. There are no current plans for either expansion or closure of the program. It lost about $50,000 last year. The actual cost for the program is approximately $47 per day per resident. Thus the program is currently losing more than $20 a day on the SSI residents and somewhat less on its one private-pay resident. Green Acres Apartments pays a $1,600 maintenance fee to the housing co-op each month. The housing cost alone is about $200 per month per resident plus utilities. The program is seen as a "mission-driven" component of the agency and has received strong support from the agency's board. The agency's strong financial position, which is sustained by larger programs that generate surpluses, has neither produced pressures to close the program nor to cut operating costs. "If someone were to wave a magic wand and raise the SSI payment from $27 to $40, I'd jump on the table and consider expanding," said the agency's director. However, the agency is in the process of developing a joint venture to construct a strictly private-pay assisted living complex that will have 120 units, including accommodation of thirty Alzheimer's patients. The agency and its partner have formed a separate for-profit corporation and have begun to evaluate sites. The new project is acknowledged as a "mission-dissonant" venture by the agency's management, but the management believes that some of the expected surplus could be reinvested in expanding access to attractive enriched housing for SSI recipients.

OPERATIONS

The program's small size is both a strength and a weakness operationally. Though it offers a homelike environment, it has all the limitations of sharing a small apartment. Although all of the staff enjoy the residents and look forward to seeing them each day, sometimes the demands are overwhelming. The inevitable aging in place of some residents raised concerns of state inspectors. The personal care aide who helps prepare meals for the residents must sometimes stop to address the needs of one of the residents who have problems with bowel and bladder control. In an attempt to address these kinds of concerns, a registered nurse was placed in charge of overseeing the medications of residents. The agency allocates one hour a week for her time to perform that function, which has given her more than a few sleepless nights. By licensure definitions, residents in an enriched housing setting must be able to self-medicate. Adult homes and enriched housing programs push the envelope. That is certainly the case for most of the residents in Green Acres Apartments. The medications of six of the eight include psychotropics. There is no formalized activities program, and the residents complain that they would like more activities and trips. The facility's size limits the staff and thus the choices residents have.

Responding to the Demands of Assisted Living

PROVIDING A HOME, CHOICE, AND A PLACE TO GROW OLD

Each resident has a private bedroom. Both residents and the personal care aides described it as a "home." As one resident said, "I got depressed and was admitted to a hospital and then to Crestview [an adult home]. Then I came here. There is no comparison. Here I have my own room." one resident said. Another said, "I'm ninety-six. I didn't expect anything, but this is more like a home. I was in an adult home with seventy-six people. Some were very disruptive." One of the aides concurred: "I want to be here when I get older. It's like being at home. Sure, they want shrimp and lobster. When they tell me that, I just have to laugh. I look forward and feel good about coming here in the morning. I thank the Lord."

Residents, however, want more choice in food and activities. The size of the facility, of course, limits their options. "What I miss is the ability to cook the way I like," one said. "I was a healthy cook and I eat lots of vegetables. The food here stinks. The other aide knew how to cook matzo balls but was not certified for assisting with medications."

The noninstitutional nature of enriched housing limits the degree of control staff can exercise over residents even if they wish to do so. Risk taking is an ongoing concern of the agency. "The phones ring a lot," the administrator responsible for the program said. "One resident wanted to go down into the city to do some shopping. We spoke to her, to her daughter, to the residents, but she went, causing everyone to worry when she returned late. The philosophy is that residents should be allowed to make choices and that, as much as possible, by assigning staff to go with them, etc., those choices should be honored but assisted in such a way as to make them as safe as possible."

"Residents are adults, and there are no prohibitions with regard to sex. It is not an issue yet," a staff member said. "A love triangle appears to be forming between one of the male residents and two of the women who are constantly fighting," the care coordinator said.

There are limits to what this program can accommodate. The program currently lacks twenty-four-hour care. It is struggling with trying to find placement or an adequate accommodation for two residents who are cognitively impaired and incontinent. "It is not the end all and be all in terms of aging in place," an administrator says. There is no wheelchair accessibility, and there are safety issues with incontinence that cannot be self-managed.

It is also a very tight living arrangement, which makes it difficult to accommodate individual personal care staff without impinging on the other residents. The more cognitively intact residents complain. Currently, an aide provides two incontinent and cognitively impaired residents additional assistance in the morning and evening. The other residents are not happy sharing the apartment with the two incontinent residents, particularly sharing the bathroom. "It looks like a nursing home here. They should be told to leave," one said. Another felt that was a cruel thing to say.

ASSURING SAFETY AND HIGH STANDARDS OF CARE

According to the administrator, "Quality of services is the mantra of this agency, and I would not be concerned about the impact of not being licensed. It would be foolish, however, for the state to select that option. Registering is nothing more than paper-pushing."

One of the difficulties in assuring safety and a high standard of care for this program is the diversity of the residents' needs. "The care needs vary," the care coordinator observed. "Some are completely independent, some cognitively impaired. They range in age from sixty to ninety-five." The facility has attempted to adapt to sicker residents. However, as the care coordinator noted, "a lot of things were falling through the cracks in terms of the old arrangements with home health aides. There were too many problems, and it was too expensive."

The organization of services is complex for such a small program. One staff member is responsible for overseeing the direct care services to the residents, one for clinical care, and another for the general maintenance of the apartments. The person responsible for personal care and the one responsible for clinical care have responsibilities for the much larger residential care program for those with developmental disabilities.

"We recently got involved in hiring care aides rather relying on the home health agency," the nursing director said. "It was clear that some of the residents could not self-medicate." Nursing now provides one hour a week to supervise this process. "There is not enough time, and it is a responsibility that gives me sleepless nights," the nursing director said. The tension between the views of registered nurses about how things should work and the actual operations of assisted living facilities is a recurring theme in almost all facilities we visited. Much of the nurse's time with the program at Green Acres involved reviewing charts and medication sheets and trying to refine the system. The problem of other residents' acceptance of those who are aging in place seemed in this case to have more to do with the care provided than with a willingness to accept residents with more serious problems. Some of the residents were more frightened for than dismissive of the residents with problems.

Farm Home
Business Strategy

MARKET NICHE

Farm Home is a large licensed adult home with a majority of residents who are state psychiatric hospital discharges. It serves as a suitable example to end this review of the diverse facilities where assisted living takes place, tying together and updating all the strands of the history of care for the frail elderly presented in Chapter 2. Because of that role in this review, I will spend a little more time setting the stage.

Farm Home is located in a small town in an insular exurban area. "If you didn't draw your first breath here, you don't belong," observed one of the staff at the facility who had moved to town more than twenty years ago and still considers herself an outsider. A sharp division persists between the "hill people," who reside higher up on the hillside and trace their families to those who raised cattle and farmed the land in the nineteenth century, and the "river rats," whose families worked in the mills or ran the ferries on the river. Two Catholic churches, both two-thirds empty and financially struggling, remain as proof that even common religious faith cannot bridge this historical social class divide.

Yet even with the division, many remain proud of the community's common history as the home of craftsmen who manufactured weapons used in the Revolutionary War and who worked in the mills that manufactured uniforms for the Union soldiers in the Civil War and the factories that made bricks used in the construction of the Empire State Building and the Rockefeller Center. The town's industry, however, died a slow death, never recovering from the Great Depression.

Ironically, given the community's past contributions to liberty, its major current industry is imprisonment. The major source of employment for local residents is overseeing true outsiders—prison inmates, mostly from New York City. A state psychiatric hospital opened nearby around 1900 and by 1960 had almost one thousand acres under cultivation. The inmates produced crops worth more than $175,000 each year. All of these lands have since been converted to a new crop, prisoners. A complex of prisons now occupies the previously cultivated land. The only community hospital serving the town closed in the early 1990s. As one local resident observed, "There was a lot of upset about the hospital's closing, but in a town that can no longer support a movie theater, how can you support a hospital?" In the process of changing to a local economy dependent on prisoners, the town has become associated with the stigma of its charges. The local economy is stagnant, and many of the citizens are dispirited.

Only in such a dispirited small community could a large facility catering to discharged psychiatric patients have been developed without meeting major local resistance. Farm Home opened in the early 1970s as a health-related facility. It concentrated on serving those discharged from the state psychiatric system, which was undergoing a massive deinstitutionalization process. The facility absorbed discharges from several state hospitals that were closing. Neither the facility's operators nor the town were prepared to manage this influx. The facility's residents were found walking naked downtown, disrupting local places of business, and frightening local citizens with their bizarre behavior. The facility is still paying a price for those early disruptive years. Anyone who is homeless, acting bizarrely, or poorly dressed is assumed to be one of Farm Home's residents. When the Farm Home staff receive calls from the mayor asking them to pick up a homeless person, it is difficult for them to convince him that the person is not one of their residents. Since the conventional wisdom in the town is that psychiatric disorders and homelessness are conditions that afflict outsiders, the mentally disabled and the homeless are all assumed to be the facility's residents.

The current owner, having worked in the adult home business in New York City during the 1980s, purchased the facility a decade ago. The median age of residents is now between sixty-five and seventy, about two thirds are male, and 70% have a psychiatric treatment history. The facility operates at close to 100% occupancy, but the waiting list of ten to fifteen applicants that it used to have has disappeared. It has a good reputation among those planning disposition in psychiatric units of state hospitals and acute hospitals in New York City. The majority of residents come from those hospitals. The skilled nursing home nearby is only about half full, and another one is being built almost next door to Farm Home. Just as the private-pay assisted living facilities in New York City worry about the low-occupancy nursing homes, the administrator of Farm Home worries that the nursing homes in his service area could draw away frail elderly admissions to his facility. The facility also faces competition for mentally disabled admissions from family care homes, which need not be licensed as adult homes if they take fewer than five residents, and the community resident programs set up by the state for former state psychiatric hospital patients, which permit the commingling of SSI and Medicaid dollars. Some of the community resident programs are owned and operated by the state, and some are contracted to nonprofit providers. Since so many of Farm Home's residents with a psychiatric history have little connection with families and communities and relatively few of its residents come from the local area, the facility does not have the typical service area characteristics of a local care provider; as a result, the owner acknowledges, the facility competes with facilities from the entire downstate area. The facility manages well with a mixed population of about 30% elderly residents and 70% somewhat younger residents with a psychiatric history. We saw a number of younger male residents assisting older, frailer residents walking. We were told that such friendships and assistance are common. The owner bristles at the idea of having adult homes with psychiatric residents being classified differently from those providing care only to the elderly, a measure included in legislation recently proposed by the governor. He predicts that it would create a housing crisis for the mentally disabled.

FINANCING

SSI pays for about 90% of the facility's residents. The "private-pay" residents have some limited Social Security and retirement benefits. There are ten private rooms allocated to the private-pay residents, and the rest are semiprivate rooms with their own bathrooms. SSI delays payment a month after one is found eligible, so the facility often has to absorb the cost of the first month, and the facility averages about six to eight new residents a month. Like other facilities, it receives only $27 per day in SSI payments, and like other facilities with limited income, it is a penny-pinching operation. Nevertheless, the facilities and programs look remarkably similar to the private facilities.

Farm Home, unlike the other facilities we looked at, can supplement its own programs for residents with state-supported services provided to the mentally ill that are not available to those in elderly-only facilities. A local public program provides for trips to ball games and other events. The local veterans groups volunteer transportation. The public mental health program provides day programs and transportation for about thirty of the residents each day who choose to participate. The local public mental health program also provides an on-site satellite center that is staffed with two social workers, two caseworkers, and one full-time and one part-time registered nurse and a part-time psychiatrist. They run groups, do counseling and crisis intervention, monitor the medication of residents, etc. The facility is also eligible for approximately $200 to $300 per resident in supportive case management funds that can be used to assist residents with incidental needs such as clothing. With this assistance, the owner-operator is able to make a modest profit on the operation.

OPERATIONS

The personal care aides assist with medication, bathing, dressing, and toileting. There are typically two aides on each shift. There are about 195 residents. All of the residents require assistance with self-medication, 70% need help with bathing, 50% with dressing, and 5% with toileting. In most cases, since this is a relatively young and physically healthy population, that assistance would appear to require relatively little time and involves mostly just cueing. Only 10% of the residents are currently receiving home care, and only 3% use a walker or other ambulatory aid. The medication assistance represents the major weak link acknowledged both by the aides we talked with and the owner. Medications are typically administered at mealtime, and residents are expected to attend all three meals.

Aides receive $7.00 an hour. The pay was the major complaint the aides we spoke with had about the job, which otherwise they regard as manageable. One is a single mother supporting three children who cannot afford the optional health insurance benefit package the facility offers, and Medicaid covers the cost of her children's health care.

In spite of all these limitations, the facility as a whole is attractive and has made a serious effort to soften the institutional character of the building. The activities programs, including the off-site programs supported by the county, in-house activities, and particularly the various groups and counseling offered by the mental health program satellite, are richer, more varied, and better than any of the programs offered by almost any of the other facilities we visited. The facility has adapted well to its surroundings and makes a profit.

Responding to the Demands of Assisted Living

Farm Home has recently renovated its dining area. Rooms are attractive and clean and compare well in appearance to low-end private-pay adult homes and unlicensed assisted living facilities. The grounds have well-maintained flower beds. The facility is a short distance from a bakery, which has become part of the daily routine of many residents. The downtown stores and library are within walking distance. This sets the facility apart from most adult homes with a large mental health population, which tend to be located in more isolated and rural locations to avoid the opposition of neighbors.

The characteristics of this home that make it similar to other mental health facilities are smoking (all the residents smoke, and most observe the facility rules that allow smoking only in the areas designated on each floor and outside the entrance); shabby, ill-fitting clothing worn by the residents (most of their SSI allowances go to pay for cigarettes); and a history of poor dental care among the residents.

Risk sharing for the frail elderly in this setting has been strongly influenced by the long legal battles over the rights of the mentally ill and the growing protections against involuntary commitments. Some residents objected to a TV monitoring system that has recently been installed in the hallways and entrances, which they consider an invasion of their privacy. Several Alzheimer's patients have ankle bracelets, which set off an alarm if they leave the building. For the others, persuasion helps, as well as offering options such as escorts for trips. If all these efforts fail, the facility and the mental health unit simply document their efforts and hope for the best. Family members and adult children, because they either live far away or are no longer connected to the residents, play no part in this process. The facility's physician has office visits on the premises twice a week. The mental health program is on site seven days a week.

Residents are aging in place. Some have outlasted all of the facility's many previous owners, living at the home almost all of its twenty-six-year life. The facility is applying for a limited home health agency license so that Medicaid can be billed directly for the additional services that are needed. As with other adult homes included in our case studies, this will allow the facility to hire additional personal care staff, probably provide more continuity and integration of care, and certainly improve the operating margin.

More than any other home, this one encapsulates all the tensions in the long history of efforts to reinvent care. A recent legislative proposal by the governor would designate facilities such as this one with a high proportion of mentally ill residents as "Mental Health Residences for Adults." The Medicaid program would then invest more resources in the adult homes catering exclusively to the elderly to try to prevent or delay nursing home admissions. In a sense, this proposal revives the nineteenth-century struggle to provide separate residential settings for the mentally ill. For Farm Home at the beginning of the twenty-first century, this separation seems less appropriate. As its administrator asks, Why should those with a mental health diagnosis not be allowed to age in place? What really distinguishes this facility's population from those with dementia? Granted, this argument does not apply to the younger mental health population and those with substance abuse problems, but what's the difference between the needs of older chronic mental health population and those of the frail, cognitively impaired elderly? Is this facility to function like the prisons next to it, as way of removing and controlling people we fear, or as a way to provide care to people within a community?

Common Lessons

Are private-market and publicly supported assisted living facilities the same? Certainly the financial picture is different. The three nonprofit public-pay facilities described in this chapter lose money, and the two owner-operated ones break even. Among those private-market assisted living facilities described in the previous chapter, all but the small nonprofit private one made a profit. The public market facilities offset their losses with endowments, private charitable giving, and additional public program dollars. Three received payments from Medicaid as ALPs, and one received additional staffing support from a state-supported mental health program. Not surprisingly, people who can afford to pay the private rates have many more attractive options, and those who can't have few.

Yet the day-to-day operations of private-pay and publicly supported assisted living have much in common. They adapt to the growing frailty of their residents in much the same way that families and NORCs do, improvising accommodations. They face the same tensions between adequate staffing and controlling costs. Most administrators of both kinds of facilities feel that they are part of a broader assisted living movement working to offer more attractive choices to consumers.

Are assisted living facilities, both private and public, accomplishing their mission? Are they providing an environment that offers the opportunity to age in place with most of the same choices and privacy one would enjoy in one's own home while at least matching the safety and standards of care of a nursing home? The answers are different for each of the ten facilities described in these two chapters. As a whole, however, these ten facilities suggest six common lessons:

1. The organization's philosophy shapes the degree of aging in place that is safely possible. Integrated delivery systems reject the notion of aging in place and restrict the degree of aging in place that is possible in their version of assisted living. Other facilities have embraced aging in place as a core value and have organized, staffed, and priced their care, as much as possible, to accommodate aging in place. The envelope has been pushed farthest by unlicensed facilities that have many of the characteristics of an adult home but neither the licensure restrictions with regard to whom they care for nor the public payment restrictions on resources. One could argue that, as more complex adaptive organizations, they are probably safer places for elderly residents, whose needs rarely fit neatly or predictably into a narrow band of services.
2. All residents and most facilities are unprepared to address the problems of aging in place. Most facilities have done a poor job of anticipating rather than reacting to the needs of their residents. They have done nothing to assist residents in dealing with the decline of their neighbors, or even to alert them ahead of time. It is hard to market decline, but the failure to prepare residents and families for it creates a backlash.
3. You get what you pay for. Homelike settings with all the amenities cost more than institutional ones. Private rooms cost more than shared ones. Public-pay adult homes are institutional settings. Adding additional funding for services to care for nursing home-eligible residents through an assisted living or Medicaid waiver program does not transform these adult homes into assisted living facilities, at least as envisioned by advocates of assisted living. With rare exceptions, all it produces is cheaper and less regulated public nursing homes.
4. Enriched housing is a closer match with the assisted living model than other licensed facilities. It provides private, noninstitutional apartment living valued by assisted living advocates and, thanks to public support for low-income housing, provides it more equally to rich and poor alike. The basic limitation of this model has to do with its inability to address the needs of the cognitively impaired.
5. There is no organizationally coherent argument for segregating care for the aging mental health population from care for the elderly population in general. One third to one half of those in assisted living facili-

ties for the elderly suffer from cognitive impairments. Most of the key medical problems in managing care for the elderly mental health population are the same problems faced in caring for the elderly in general.
6. The direct care staff are both the salvation and the Achilles' heel of assisted living. Some are remarkable persons, guardian angels with special gifts. They experience great joy in their work, but they often feel undervalued and underpaid. The bond and relationships that they form with residents is crucial. The most fundamental rule of quality of care, as the Institute of Medicine report noted, is that it has to be based on a continuous healing relationship. The personal care aides are at the core of that relationship in assisted living. Adequate staffing, decent working conditions, living wages, and appropriate recognition of personal care aides are the keys to quality of care in assisted living.

All of these facilities, both private-pay and public, have changed, addressing increasingly more complex needs as their residents age. Competition in the private-pay market has increased, and individuals with more complex medical needs are admitted to assure fill up. Most residents in licensed adult homes and enriched housing can no longer self-administer their medications. That is a technical violation of their licensure requirements that is conveniently overlooked. The ability to pay privately for care is no guarantee against substandard care, particularly as private assisted living facilities face increasingly intense price competition. Nursing home capacity is no longer expanding, and the population of frail elderly grows. As noted by many of the managers we talked with, the limited regulation and complete absence of public oversight of the look-alike unlicensed facilities may offer little in the way of a counterbalancing force against the bottom-line financial pressures faced by many. A time bomb is ticking. If not diffused, a wave of patient care problems will envelop both private-market and public-pay assisted living facilities.

How can the time bomb be defused and the promise of assisted living be realized? I will assemble all the pieces of the puzzle collected in this book and try to answer this question in its final section.

Part III
Reinventing Care

7
A Future for Care

Neither the old nor the new models of care fit well with the day-to-day realities described in the preceding section. The elderly and their families wanted less institutional settings for care and more control of their lives. Developers, seeing a growing, profitable market, constructed facilities. The Medicaid program, seeing it as a way to reduce the cost of care for nursing home patients, offered assisted living options. For the most part, however, everyone has been disappointed. Assisted living has not assured the elderly the autonomy of a homelike environment and has not given developers the profits or state Medicaid programs the savings that they sought.

While the realities of assisted living have rarely matched the rhetoric, it has shaken the foundation of the existing system of care. Many still see it as a social movement, much like the psychiatric deinstitutionalization movement that began in the 1960s but more sweeping. Its advocates challenged the purpose of care, the role of government regulation, and the existing notions about the most appropriate location of care. They argued that care should enrich rather than impoverish people's lives, that government should not be involved, and that care should be provided in people's homes rather than in institutions. Nothing will be the same again. Regulators are confused about what they should regulate, providers are uncertain about what they should be providing, and consumers are bewildered about what they are buying.

This final chapter summarizes the fragments of ideas that seem worth salvaging from this confusion. It distills from the story told in this book a crude outline of a road map for the development of a more hopeful future for care.

The Goal

The goal should be to assure a full range of choices for all those who need assisted living services in a way that maximizes their control over their lives while assuring a single standard of safety and quality of care.

The rallying cry of assisted living advocates is choice. Individuals and families should be able to choose to have care in their homes. They should be able do what they want with their own lives and take risks if they chose to do so. They should not have to move. They should be able to choose to age in place. Assisted living advocates are clearer about what they do not want than what they do want. They do not want florescent lighting and sterile asphalt tile corridors, the loss of privacy and regimens that transform customers into patients. Most developers and consumer advocates of assisted livings services speak with one voice on these concerns. They see choice as the way individuals improve their quality of life. Those facing the day-to-day problems of assisted living—of doing their job well, of deciding what to do with their aging relative, or of learning to live with their neighbors in assisted living facilities—may be impatient with such abstract, long-term goals. However, achieving the goals of freedom of choice and a single standard of care will help everyone—providers, the elderly, and their families—address all of these immediate problems.

The largest barrier to the achievement of this goal, of course, is the financial one. How do we assure choice for everyone and not simply enrich the lives of the few who are affluent enough to have choices while impoverishing the lives of everyone else?

Yet perhaps embedded in the assisted living movement is the potential for a far more fundamental shift in the paradigm of how we think about the financing and organization of such care. Such a shift is supported by the day-to-day experiences of the elderly residents of the facilities described in Part II of this book who noted that the relationships they have with staff and their fellow residents are far more important than the opulence of their surroundings. It is supported by a persuasive emerging body of research about what shapes the effectiveness of such communities and the health of their residents. The experiences of those we spoke with offer several hints about how a new model of care might be constructed.

First, assisted living organizations that work do not really work the way we conventionally think organizations that provide services should. They are more fluid, continuously adapting to the changing needs of their residents. In many ways, they exemplify how all health and social services organizations should work. The Institute of Medicine in its comprehensive review of the safety and quality of care in health settings argued that such "complex adaptive organizations" help assure a high level of safety and quality of care (Institute of Medicine 2001, 68). Mechanical systems assume that the only choices are between control and chaos. In contrast, adaptive systems acknowledge a "zone of complexity" in which there are more choices about outcomes. Assisted living lies in that zone of complexity where it is rarely clear when it is no longer acceptable for an individual to live where they do with the current services they are receiving.

Effectively functioning complex adaptive systems, as suggested in the Institute of Medicine's report on quality, include the following attributes:

- Adaptable elements: The elements of the system can change themselves. No one waits for directives from central offices or state regulators to make changes that improve the quality of life of residents.
- Simple rules: A few locally applied simple rules can respond most effectively to the diverse individual needs of residents.
- Emergent novelty: Continual creativity is the natural state of the system.
- Co-evolution: Assisted living develops and evolves through constant tension, uncertainty, and anxiety—all healthy attributes of complex adaptive systems.
- Context matters: Systems exist within systems. The community and the larger environment in which assisted living facilities operate are critical to the quality of life of residents. (adapted from Plsek 2001, 326)

The internal operations of the better assisted living facilities described in Part II of this book reflect these attributes.

Second, and perhaps more important in addressing the financial issue, assisted living facilities do not operate in a vacuum. Context matters. The quality of life in the larger community can have a greater effect on residents than the facility itself. It is this link that ties the affluent who can afford high-end private assisted living with everyone else.

In terms of context, income and wealth, more than any other factors, affect quality of life and life expectancy. The higher the income an individual has, the longer that individual can expect to live. However, when one compares life expectancies of communities and nations as a whole, per capita income ceases to be as powerful a predictor. Once per capita income passes a level necessary to assure an adequate standard of living, income disparities rather than per capita income become better predictors of life expectancy. Developed countries with lower per capita gross domestic products than the United States but less income inequality (Japan, Sweden, Iceland, Canada, and France, for example) have higher life expectancies (Wilkinson 1996). Similarly, in the United States, metropolitan areas with larger income inequalities have larger excess death rates. In fact, metropolitan areas with greater income inequality have higher mortality rates at all income levels (Lynch et al. 1998). New Yorkers, for example, have the highest per capita income in the country, but their relative income inequality is reflected in the overall poor health status of elderly New Yorkers. Relative income disparities and poverty rates influence social relationships, which in turn affect the social cohesiveness, trust, and quality of the direct care provided and, ultimately, the health of a population. The high-rise private security and personal services that are offered in affluent assisted living facilities are poor substitutes for a viable community life. As one researcher observed, the growing geographic concentration of poverty in urban areas "strains the fragile social fabric that keeps anarchy at bay and makes it possible for cities to be communities and not just agglomerations of fearful strangers" (Jargowsky 1996, 185).

Thus, if one wishes to increase the life expectancy and quality of life of the frail elderly, perhaps the best approach would be policies that reduce poverty. As noted in Chapter 1, if all the income disparities among the elderly in the New York metropolitan area were eliminated, all elderly persons in New York City could afford the expense of private-market assisted living, and there would be no need for publicly supported facilities. The average income of its elderly residents is more than $25,000 and the average net worth more than $310,000. Individuals with such a financial profile could afford even the most costly facilities. Past public policies toward the elderly in the United States suggest that it certainly doesn't take a revolution to redistribute income and reap the benefits of life expectancy increases. The introduction of Social Security in the late 1930s and the indexing of Social Security payments to inflation in the late 1960s and early 1970s were both associated with large mortality reductions among the elderly that were not reflected in younger age groups (House and Williams 2000). In addition, while life expectancy at birth in England, Sweden, France, and Japan well exceeds that of the United States, life expectancy at age eighty in the United States greatly exceeds that of these other countries (Preston and Elo 1996). One plausible explanation of the better outcomes for the elderly in the United States is that the elderly have almost universal health insurance coverage through Medicare, while younger age groups have far more fragmentary coverage than offered in these other countries. The goal of universal access to a full range of health services for the elderly has already been largely achieved. Policies that redistribute income in a way that reduces poverty rates not only expand choices but also increase life expectancy.

The Strategy

How could such an admittedly elusive, utopian goal be achieved? One could start with taking advantage of the pressures on the existing system of long-term care, the resourcefulness of complex adaptive organizations, and the beneficial effects of reducing economic disparities. Five simple rules could guide this strategy.

1. Use the forces already transforming care.

Demographic shifts, economic pressures, technological change, the changing expectations of the elderly and their families, and the resulting political pressures are already transforming care. It's a matter of taking full advantage of these forces.

The population of the United States continues to age. In New York City alone there are now more than one million individuals over the age of sixty-five and more than 139,501 individuals over the age of eighty-five (Claritas 1998). The real population pressures on services for the elderly in the United States and in New York City, however, will begin as the oldest members of the post–World War II baby boom generation reach eighty-five in 2030. The impact this will have on health care providers, community services providers, developers, politicians, and families is obvious. The existing physical and financial arrangements for care simply will not be able to sustain the explosive growth in elderly population that is to come.

The total pool of dollars now allocated to elderly care is immense and growing. The Medicaid program in New York City alone now spends almost $5 billion dollars per year, or almost $20,000 for every Medicaid-eligible person over sixty-five (see Table 1.1). The average cost for Medicare coverage for the over-sixty-five population in New York is more than $9,000 per person overall and more than 50% higher for the low-income elderly who are also eligible for Medicaid. Supplemental Security Income (SSI) payments to single elderly persons who lack other forms of income from pensions, Social Security, or other sources currently amount to $9,855 a year per person. In other words, more than $43,000 per person per year is currently being expended to maintain the "safety net floor" for the elderly in New York City who receive all of these benefits. This estimate does not include the value of the public subsidies for housing, utilities, and food stamps or the subsidies provided by private charitable groups. In addition, New York City's elderly residents have $25.3 billion in private income and $312.6 billion in private assets to support the care that they need. As the expenditures for long-term care grow, the pressure to use them more intelligently increases.

The rapid advances in medical science and information technology are also having a profound impact on the elderly and their caregivers. Already, nursing home use is declining, in part a reflection of the improved health of the elderly population (Manton and Gu 2001). New breakthroughs such as vaccinations for chronic diseases and advances in rehabilitation will continue to transform the composition of the elderly population and their care needs. A healthier elderly population will, as a result, have more choices about how and where to live. They will also have far more information on which to base those choices. With a few clicks of the mouse one can get information about the most recent inspection report and comparable measures of performance on any nursing home in the country as well as detailed information on other nursing homes in the same neighborhood. The Internet has also expanded the sources of support available to individuals and their families and has facilitated disease-specific advocacy and the diffusion of information about new therapies and forms of care. It is profoundly altering the traditional paternalistic relationship between providers and their patients. The culture of health-related care is beginning to look more like the customer-centered culture of a Hyatt or Marriott hotel.

The growth of the elderly population, the expansion of the financial resources to support them, and rapid changes in technological capacity to address their needs has changed expectations. Better-educated and more affluent elderly and their families expect to have choices and to have more control of their lives and their care. As a result, they are far less willing to be processed. These changing expectations are forcing changes in the design and organization of long-term care services.

2. Nurture complex systems.

Nurturing care settings as complex adaptive systems improves those settings' ability to respond to the individual wishes and unique needs of their residents. No two assisted living organizations are alike. Each has its own distinctive characteristics that have evolved from interactions with residents and the local community. That distinctiveness needs to be valued and preserved. Safety and quality of care can't be preserved by cookie-cutter standards.

A responsive complex system does not wait for the directives of regulators, planners, or corporate CEOs. It responds to immediate needs. Indeed, the dominant form of assisted living is informal. At least two thirds of all care is still provided by family members. Much assistance is still provided by neighbors. In urban areas naturally occurring retirement communities (NORCs) spring up. They are self-organized and evolve from the services of doormen to a full array of services. Apartment complexes and co-op housing developments have responded to the growing frailty of residents and neighbors. Similarly, licensed adult homes have responded to the needs of their residents who are aging in place by adding new services.

Patient-centered services require adapting to the distinctive and changing needs of individual residents, but this too rarely happens. Much of the care for the elderly is still organized around the needs of national long-term care corporations, regional integrated delivery systems, the professional groups providing care, and the public agencies responsible for monitoring and financing those organizations and professionals. When reality no longer fits such structures, elaborate fictions are created. Adult homes, for example, create separate limited licensed home health agencies so that the nurse whom they have hired to administer medications may do so, since facilities licensed as adult homes are prohibited from providing this service. Supply responds to financial forces that have little to do with needs, creating booms and busts and economically disenfranchising as many as two thirds of the elderly. Regulators almost inevitably focus on the things that can be easily documented and thus lose sight of the things that are most important to residents and sometimes even the things that end up in headlines in the continuing cycle of newspaper exposés.

3. Reduce economic disparities.

As noted previously, an increasingly persuasive literature in social epidemiology suggests the beneficial effects of reduced economic disparities. Income disparities shape social relationships (trust, social participation, civic virtues, social cohesiveness, solidarity, etc.). The differences in cancer and heart disease death rates are tied more to the degree of social cohesion of communities and societies than to rates of smoking and obesity. Strong and supportive social networks reduce the likelihood of admissions to hospitals and long-term care facilities. Indeed, the major advantage offered by assisted living communities is a reduction in social isolation. Social isolation and lack of cohesiveness may help explain why urban living carries with it a risk of death similar to more widely documented risk factors such as smoking or low income (House et al. 2000).

Disparities produce a "gradient effect" of poorer health, and not just poorer health for those in the lowest income group. For example, a study of British civil servants has showed that heart disease rates decline as one goes further up the civil service scale (Brunner 1996). That study and an expanding body of research results show that hierarchy negatively affects the control that individuals exercise over their immediate environment and determines the level of stress one experiences (Sapolosky 1993; Wilkinson 1996). Other studies conclude that these hierarchical stress effects can be moderated by increasing job control (e.g., workers' control over the use of skills on the job, authority to make decisions about the organization of their work, and ability to exert control over uncertainties at work) (Vahtera et al. 2000). It requires but a modest leap to suggest that similar effects are applicable to long-term care residents and their caregivers (Chipperfield et al. 1999; Mirowsky and Ross 1998). Equality, as some researchers have concluded, is good medicine (Daniels et al. 2000).

4. Swim upstream.

The description of New York City's long-term care system offered in the first chapter of this book brings to mind an often-told parable: A Good

Samaritan leaps into a flooded stream to save a drowning person floating by in the current. Not having caught his breath after the successful rescue, he leaps in again to save another. This is repeated many times before the exhausted Samaritan finally runs upstream along the bank to find out what is causing people to fall in.

The stream in the case of care for the elderly is the traditional continuum of care, which moves the frail elderly into increasingly costly and more formalized settings as they become less able to care for themselves. Many people slip further down this stream needlessly. Most individuals would prefer to age in place, and most of the evidence regarding transfer trauma and the importance of maintaining social support networks confirm the wisdom of such preferences. The reasons most people relocate to assisted living facilities involve concerns about personal security and social isolation. Inadequate housing, unsafe neighborhoods, and the loss of spouses and friends increase the likelihood of such relocations. Many transfers to nursing homes take place not because medical and personal care needs can no longer be met where the person is but because they can no longer be afforded.

In addition, aging in place does not work when it impinges on the quality of life of neighbors or other facility residents. This factor preventing aging in place is in part a result of failures in design and planning. Facilities must make accommodations in their physical design, in their staffing, and in how they prepare residents for the deteriorating condition of others. The more a facility can design and plan for the eventualities of aging in place, the less likelihood that the environment for other residents will be degraded by the process.

The further one is swept down the continuum-of-care stream, the less choice and control one has as a recipient or as a provider of care, and the more stressful and, consequently, unhealthy the situation is for both. Individual risk contracts in the form of documents negotiated among facilities, residents, and family members that exempt providers from responsibility for what a resident chooses to do against a facility's best judgment rarely exist. They are mostly a fantasy advocated by lawyers for the assisted living industry. The true risk contracts are implied by an individual's choice of location of care. If one chooses to receive care at home, it implies an assumption of risk that is never present in an assisted living facility. Even where a philosophy of resident control is officially espoused, frontline care providers will not permit risky choices.

Thus the only way an elderly person can be assured of control is to be cared for in his or her own home. If you own your home, you have the greatest choice over what you do with it and how you live within it. If you rent, you have less. If you choose to live in an assisted living community you forgo rights even as a tenant of a rental property, and you relinquished all management rights to the facility. There is rarely any pretense, however, that real control within an assisted living facility is exercised by anyone other than its operators and owners. While most facilities take advantage of resident councils to get feedback on how well they are doing, there is little pretense of resident governance. Few so-called resident councils have officers, and most are convened and directed by the facility's management. Operators take for granted that they have control.

The upstream informal care system still provides most of the direct care for the frail elderly in the United States. Most assisted living takes place in people's homes, where the aging person or family members organize it. A "midrange" estimate places the number of informal caregivers nationally at 25.8 million and the total value of their services at $196 billion, almost twice the amount spent nationally for nursing home and home care services (Arno and Levine 1999). In addition, much of the formal care is not managed and controlled by the operators of assisted living or long-term care facilities. Just as assisted living facilities negotiate contracts with home health agencies and other providers, so do the elderly and their families.

5. Increase resident ownership.

Once one enters the formal care system, without ownership or even the rights of a tenant, one loses control. One has no choice in the transactions that take place in publicly traded national chains that buy and sell off facilities with amazing rapidity, using the occupants as assets in these transactions. Nor do the forays of local nonprofit and for-profit hospital-based integrated delivery systems into the assisted living market provide much more assurance of control. Assisted living becomes a narrow circumscribed feeder to other parts of such systems, thus explicitly contradicting the notion of aging in place. Moreover, such systems are far from immune to the mergers and divestitures typically associated with the publicly traded national chains.

Of course ownership isn't everything. The ultimate test of control, of course, is not ownership but choice. Some may choose short-term commitments of renting rather than owning. Some may wish to forgo the rights of tenancy for the services and security offered by assisted living communities. Some may not even wish to age in place. As the stories in this book have shown, the private market has proved far more aggressive and responsive in recognizing and filling the growing demand for such choices than nonprofit integrated delivery systems. Markets and choice work best when there is real competition and complete information. Prospective residents and their families, however, have to know what they are buying and that clear standards are enforced. The growth of assisted living reflects the growing power of consumers. Powerful consumers usually insist on having services organized around them. The powerless consumers are the ones processed on an assembly line at the convenience of the specialists who attend to their care. The childbirth education and hospice movements pointed the way. Those movements transformed the birth and death experiences of families. The assisted living movement will do the same for long-term care.

The struggle to provide assisted living for the indigent parallels the longer-term struggle to provide decent affordable housing to low-income persons. What has been learned in the latter may offer some guidance for the former. There has been a growing disillusionment both with public housing and the ability of nonprofit groups to fill the low-income housing void (Salinas and Mildner 1992). State and federal policy has moved toward more emphasis on efforts to support private-sector housing for low-income families through subsidies. While opinions differ about the extent of the subsidies, there is a widespread consensus across the political spectrum on the nature of the change that is needed. Currently, about 2.4 million low-income households receive federal Section 8 housing subsidies; 1.4 million of these households receive vouchers that make up the difference between 30% of the household income and the going market rental rates in the private unsubsidized housing market ("A Modest Boost" 1998). While nationally this voucher program has not been budgeted at a level to fully meet the need for such support, the quality of the housing stock for low-income families has improved, and income disparities in housing have declined over the last two decades (Orr and Peach 1999; "State of the Nation's Low-Income Housing" 1999).

The shift in housing policy parallels some ideas of the Medicaid consumer account program approach advocated by the Assisted Living Federation of America (ALFA). It proposes using state Medicaid funds to support a similar voucher program for low-income individuals in need of long-term care services (Assisted Living Federation of America 2000). The proposal argues for the creation of a "level playing field" for all organizations that provide assisted living (e.g., nursing homes, assisted living, home care, etc.) by creating an account for each person and allowing the consumer to choose how to use it. To prevent providers from simply using such a program as a way to raise their prices, the program would have to provide full payment for the care offered; that is, providers who would charge more than the program would allow would not be eligible. Ideally, this would also provide a level playing field for indigent individuals seeking assisted living care, giving them essentially the same power in the market as private-pay assisted living consumers.

Yet by far the strongest theme in housing policy and research is not so much the relative efficiency of the private housing market but the value of home ownership. The values the assisted living movement champions are autonomy and control, which are maximized by home ownership.

Tactics

I have described the goal and summarized the strategy with five simple rules: (1) use the forces already transforming care, (2) nurture complex systems, (3) address social and economic disparities, (4) move upstream, and (5) encourage consumer ownership. How do people and organizations implement the strategy? Tactics involve moving people and organizations over terrain. In order to change a system, you have to be thoroughly familiar with the terrain, or how the existing system works. I now suggest five simple rules for guiding tactics within the existing system based on the findings that have been described in this book.

1. Couch the debate in terms of a consumer rebellion.

Saying it is a consumer rebellion helps make it one and takes advantage of all the promotional rhetoric of the industry. As all developers understand, the last thing any elderly person wants is to move to a nursing home. This would be true even without the bad press about nursing homes that influenced the public's perceptions for decades. People resist being uprooted from their homes and familiar surroundings. They want to age in place and maintain as much of their freedom as possible. Most of the research evidence suggests that these attitudes are healthy and should be encouraged. Other things being equal, people live longer and stay healthier living where they have always lived and doing what they have always enjoyed doing. As shown in the review of the transfer trauma literature in Chapter 3, relocation, on the whole, seems to worsen the health of the frail elderly and increase their chances of death.

Most people with sufficient resources prefer to age in place and, as much as possible, sustain their freedom and independence in familiar surroundings to the end. Successful developers, operators, and community relations directors know what sells and have done a good job selling it. "This is not a nursing home," they reassure their prospective tenants. "This is your home, and we will respect your freedom and independence. If you are like most of our residents, you will never have to go through the trauma of moving again."

It is an effective sales pitch but one that shades the truth. Few assisted living communities seriously embrace the notion of aging in place. A survey of Kansas facilities found that, because of funding and staffing constraints, most had admission and discharge policies that were more restrictive than state regulations required (Chapin and Dobbs-Kepper 2001). Similarly, our survey of licensed facilities in New York State found little flexibility in discharge policies. The two assisted living facilities described in the preceding chapters that were components of integrated delivery systems restricted their residents to those with few medical or personal care needs.

Choice is also more limited than it would be in one's home. As the residents we talked with indicated, an assisted living facility is not a home. Meals follow a schedule, and one's freedom is limited by the needs of other community members, whose lives become more intertwined with one's own than do one's neighbors in one's own home.

While most residents like the idea of aging in place for themselves, assisted living communities have done a poor job of preparing residents to deal with the aging in place of others. The residents we talked with expressed anger and frustration about the growing frailty and cognitive impairment they saw around them. "This is becoming a nursing home," some said. They found the cognitive rather than the physical impairments of other residents the most difficult to deal with, perhaps because it heightened their sense of isolation and fear.

Regulations governing licensure and liability set limits on how much risk facilities can take. If for no other reason, facilities need liability insurance coverage to satisfy their financial backers, and that coverage comes with conditions that restrict the risks that facilities can assume. As a consequence, the degree of aging in place that is acceptable is limited. Facilities may push the envelope a bit, but a true assisted living consumer rebellion can never achieve its goals in an organized institutional setting.

2. Encourage greater resident income integration within facilities.

Developers and operators will do whatever is profitable. While in New York State there is an almost complete separation between assisted living facilities providing care to private-pay residents and those providing care to indigent residents, little of the same separation exists in nursing homes. The state's relatively high Medicaid nursing home payment rates explain the difference. In 1999 those payments contributed to $159 million in profits for New York City's 161 nursing homes, and comparable profits have been sustained for the last five years (New York State Department of Health 2001a).

Reflecting the differences in profitability, there is growing excess capacity in the private-market assisted living sector and shortages of comparable quality arrangements for public-pay clients. Private-market assisted living developers anticipate returns on their investment as high as 40%. In contrast, public-pay assisted living facilities providing a good standard of care sometimes struggle to find ways to make up losses as high as 40%. Their major source of income is SSI payments provided to indigent residents. SSI provides $27 a day to cover room, board, and some personal care services. It costs an average of $48 to board a dog in Manhattan, which is roughly the same as what some of the assisted living providers we interviewed said were their costs. A few of the more fortunate nonprofits have sufficient charitable donations or endowments to fill the gap. Some have been able to take advantage of the state's assisted living program that provides additional Medicaid payments for nursing home–eligible residents. Others have been able to enrich their services with state-supported services for the mentally ill. Still others have been able to get Medicaid funds through the creation of limited-license home health agencies. Most must make do as best they can. A few, of course, become the subject of headlines that highlight substandard care and abuses. The differences in revenues produce stark differences in both supply and quality.

Given the large Medicaid expenditures for nursing home care and other health services and the excess capacity in the private assisted living sector, modest increases in public payments could produce expanded public use of private-pay assisted living facilities. While many private assisted living facilities offer discounts to prospective customers in order to increase occupancy, several operators freely acknowledged the practice of transferring first-day-eligible Medicaid recipients to nursing homes. Yet Medicaid nursing home care can cost up to five times as much as assisted living care. Expanded public spending for assisted living care would be a more efficient use of public funds.

3. Focus on the needs of direct care providers.

The bricks and mortar of facilities are ultimately of little importance. As in other long-term care settings, those who provide the direct care in assisted living facilities make all the difference. The residents I talked with were most likely to mention the relationship they had with their caregivers either as what they liked most about where they lived or as a source of complaints. "The key to quality of care for our residents is recruiting and retaining quality staff," providers say (McGurk 2000, 2). Certainly no adult child who has tried to organize in-home services for a parent would disagree.

The trusting relationships that are often formed between caregivers and residents are also an import source of satisfaction among staff. In spite of generally lower pay, the turnover of personal care aides tends to be lower in assisted living facilities than in nursing homes. "It's like being at home, and we are like family," one aide said. The degree of control and the extent and richness of the interaction with residents make working in an assisted living environment more enjoyable than similar work in hospitals or nursing homes. It is the long-term care equivalent of the maternity floor in a hospital, which has long been the assignment most desired by most nursing staff.

Nevertheless, like all long-term care providers, assisted living facilities face a staffing crisis. The nursing home industry has an average annual turnover rate of 93% for its direct care workers, compared with an overall United States labor market average turnover rate of 10% (McGurk 2000, 3). Annual turnover rates are 79% among assisted living "universal workers"—direct care staff who provide not only personal care services but also housekeeping and meal services (Christianson 1998, 1–2).

"Especially in an economy with low unemployment, it is easier for potential direct care workers to find work in less demanding and higher paying jobs.... The work is physically and emotionally demanding, the hours are long, the wages are low compared to the work required, and unfortunately, many facilities have not offered benefits in the past," an industry report observed (McGurk 2000, 2). "I've been here two years and get $7.00 an hour with no benefits. I have three children I support by myself, and I need more money for my family," one direct care worker told me. One aide in New York City who sees no future in her job and plans to reenter the military to become a nurse said, "When I was responsible for one person [as a home care aide], I got $7.00 an hour. Now I am responsible for sixteen people and get $7.50." Another aide said, "I want to provide the same care I want to receive when I grow old, but I also know that the best I'll be able to afford wouldn't get me space in the parking lot of this facility!"

I also heard examples of the difficult working conditions aides can find themselves in, such as working short staffed; working as a "universal worker" on weekends, nights, or when other staff are out; and the empowerment of residents at the expense of the exploitation of their direct care providers. At two facilities, when the resident population goes down, direct care staff hours are cut. One aide, the only male employee at his facility, had to leave because he was no longer working full time. Many direct care workers spoke of the difficulties connected with watching residents they have bonded with deteriorate.

Without sufficient respect, working conditions, and pay for direct care providers, no improvements will be possible.

4. Push for more effective public regulation and enforcement.

The dance of regulation requires skillful choreography to set standards for care and safety. No one would be willing to invest in stocks or fly on a commercial airline without the assurances and confidence that public regulation provides. Why should elderly individuals trust their money and lives to an assisted living facility without similar oversight?

Facility operators, however, are reluctant to dance. At every state and national association meeting, private industry operators tell their peers, "If we don't address the problem of providing adequate information to consumers and assuring standards of safety and quality, the government will." Yet they resist. They resist the additional burden. They fear the restrictions on their ability to innovate. The jobs and incomes of individuals are on the line. Admissions directors must meet their quotas. Facility managers must achieve occupancy targets and keep expenses under budget. Operators must meet the expectations of owners and stockholders.

State regulators are also reluctant to regulate exclusively private-market assisted living. Their first responsibility is to provide oversight for facilities that care for residents supported by public dollars. Inspections of Medicaid- and Medicare-supported facilities are subsidized with federal dollars. No similar subsidies exist for the inspection of private assisted living facilities. Even for the federally mandated and subsidized inspections of nursing homes, the staffing is inadequate and the turnover of inspectors high. Expanding the responsibilities of state licensure agencies faced with budget constraints spreads the staff even thinner.

Some assisted living developers argue that the government has no more business regulating private-pay assisted living than it does regulating the care one chooses to pay for privately in one's own home. Assisted living facilities that provide residents their own apartments, which they can furnish any way they choose, certainly look like homes. However, this argument doesn't hold up under closer inspection. The widely copied model admission agreement that ALFA has provided as a guide to the industry suggests something else:

> The Community may terminate this Agreement at any time, with or without cause, by giving thirty (30) days written notice to You and to Your responsible person, if applicable. In addition, it is the policy of the Community to terminate for reasons including, but not be limited to, the following: Your failure to pay the Basic Services Rate or additional charges for services You have requested within ten (10) days of the due date; Your failure to comply with State or local law after receiving written notice of the alleged violation; Your failure to comply with the Community's Rules and Regulations . . . ; a change in the use of the Community; or a finding by the Community that the Community is inappropriate for Your care. Notwithstanding the foregoing, the Community may terminate this Agreement at any time by giving You (fill in desired notice provision) days written notice if You are engaging in behavior which is a threat to the mental and/or physical health or safety of You or to the mental and/or physical safety of others in the Community. . . .
>
> This Agreement gives You the right to live in the Community and to

have as much freedom and choice regarding your life here as possible. However, it does not give You the rights of a "tenant" as state law defines that term. The Community reserves the sole right to provide management of the Community in the best interests of all Residents and reserves the right to manage or make all decisions concerning the admission, terms of admission or dismissal of other Residents consistent with state law. (Assisted Living Federation of America 1999, 8, 9)

A residence where one lacks the basic rights of a tenant and can be removed without cause with thirty days' notice or a shorter period if the "Community" concludes that his or her behavior threatens the mental health and physical safety of himself or herself or other residents is not a private home. The "Community" under such conditions assumes responsibilities for the health and safety of residents beyond that of a landlord, and residents cede control over the conduct of their lives in ways that they would not in their own home. There is nothing wrong with such contracts, and they are probably essential for the safe operation of most assisted living facilities. However, under such arrangements the facility assumes the same responsibilities for the health and safety of residents as a health-related facility and therefore should be licensed, regulated, and inspected as such. Insistence on these standards for private assisted living would also facilitate greater income integration of facility residents by eliminating the ability of exclusively private-pay facilities to circumvent public regulation.

In New York City, at least, tenants have rights not offered to residents of assisted living facilities. This was brought home to me in a visit to the Manhattan Westside Atria, a luxuriously refurbished residential hotel complete with parlors, gas fireplaces, a penthouse cappuccino bar, and gardens with a view of the Manhattan skyline. I was discussing the decision to discharge residents no longer safely able to live with the degree of independence the facility required. The home health agency under contract with the facility made the decision regarding discharge, and the arrangements for discharge were carried out as quickly as possible. "Oh, we also have tenants though," the community relations director said. The facility houses 166 assisted living residents, and interspersed on the floors with the apartments of the residents are units occupied by seventy-seven tenants who predate the conversion of the building to an assisted living facility. It is, as a result, perhaps one of the only age-integrated assisted living facilities in the country. The age distribution is more like that of the NORC apartment complexes in the city, and there are even a few families with young children.

5. Expand the definition of assisted living to include NORCs.

Housing in most cities includes a complex network of naturally occurring assisted living developments or NORCs. They are concentrations of individuals who are aging in place and have responded in many of the same ways that many assisted living facilities have to the aging of their residents. The tenant associations in those NORCs have hired service coordinators and offered space in exchange for free services to home health agencies and satellite-based practices. They have senior center activities and day care programs. Indeed some of the older look-alikes or unlicensed assisted living facilities have evolved in much the same way. They started out as residential hotels and then added services. Some, such as the Esplanade in Manhattan, part of a family-run operation that has provided residential hotel services for seniors for more than forty years, now has a full range of services and even offers care for Alzheimer's residents:

> Hearthstone at the Esplanade, New York is located in the heart of New York City in Manhattan's Upper West Side. On the 7th floor of one of New York's most eminent and well-established Assisted Living Residences, the Residence feels like a large traditional New York apartment. On the Hearthstone Floor are an elegant dining room and kitchen with a hearth, a library/piano room, and a special six-person Enhanced Life area with its own living and dining room and view of the Hudson River.
>
> Riverside Park, one of the world's largest urban parks, is located one block away and provides a place for frequent accompanied walks for residents. The artistic and performance community of New York also provides a link to the community for residents who either go to the theatre accompanied by Hearthstone staff, or as performers come to Hearthstone at the Esplanade to perform. (Hearthstone 2002)

The decision to expand the offering of such services was a response to the needs of residents and their families. Similar expansion plans are under way in other private-pay licensed and unlicensed facilities.

The boundaries between these developments and those developed by tenant associations and the boards of co-ops are blurred. Some NORCs now offer an array of services similar to the formally developed assisted living projects at a fraction of the cost. They adhere to the "philosophy" of the assisted living movement better than most of the developers who claim to espouse it. The residences are people's homes, not just homelike environments. They exist because people have indeed aged in place. People have the choice to stay in a setting where they have a maximum degree of independence.

NORCs' natural evolution into organized care, however, gives them two distinct advantages. First, they offer a way to avoid the stigma that even the most graciously designed assisted living facilities suffer from. As a longtime advocate of this model explained, "The goal is to engage people before they need help. The senior center and activities programs organized by the co-ops and apartment complexes provide a link to younger seniors and a familiar place to go when they need help without being labeled. Unlike most assisted living arrangements, it is proactive, not a reactive response to an emergency." That is the essence of the "continuous healing relationship" that the recent Institute of Medicine report identified as one of the keys to high-quality care in the twenty-first century (Institute of Medicine 2001). Second, NORCs moderate the concern of assisted living residents about their aging neighbors, who are reminders of their own mortality. The advantage that NORCs have is that those reminders come in the form of neighbors and friends with whom they have lived for forty years or more. They are not intruding strangers as they often are in assisted living facilities.

The NORCs and other family- or community-based arrangements are the embodiment of what consumers say they want. Assisted living developments are but a pale reflection of these preferences.

Common Bonds

Arlo Guthrie, son of folk singer Woody Guthrie, who spent his last years in Creedmoor State Hospital in Queens, once advocated the creation of an "un–neutron bomb." Unlike the neutron bomb that destroys people and leaves the buildings standing, the un–neutron bomb would save the people and destroy the buildings. That is my conclusion about how to advance the assisted living consumer movement to the next level. The assisted living movement urges that the frail elderly should (1) age in place, (2) preserve their autonomy wherever possible, and (3) live in a supportive, homelike environment. Furthermore, just as with other forms of deinstitutionalization, a good deal of cross-cultural and epidemiological evidence shows that it enhances the length and the quality of lives. The essence of the strategy and tactics described in this final chapter is two-pronged:

- Aggressively promote the naturally occurring models of assisted living as the options that are most compatible with the goals and values of assisted living movement. Family- and community-based assisted living and the NORCs that develop in neighborhoods allow individuals to age in place in age-integrated environments that maximize their autonomy. NORCs are the only affordable option for most and are well suited to urban apartment living settings, where there are growing natural concentrations of frail elderly.

- Demand and aggressively seek a single standard of assisted living licensure for all senior housing and residential facilities that seek to limit or abridge the normal rights of tenants. This, not who is paying the bill, is the "line in the sand" that distinguishes homes from institutions that require licensure and regulation. Licensure should require at a minimum full disclosure of the ownership and some fair share arrangement to provide units for low-income residents. Regulations should support the greatest degree of aging in place, autonomy, and risk taking that is feasible. Assisted living is a complex adaptive system that shares a common purpose and adheres to simple rules to guide development whether as part of the informal or the formal institutional system.

Goals are achieved, of course, not because of strategy and tactics. They are achieved if they can marshal the financing and the committed foot soldiers. The jaded—and no one who has worked or received care in long-term care settings is not at least a little bit jaded—will be skeptical about what I have proposed. Of course, the Devil (or at least the rich array of very powerful special interests) lurks in the details. The key to success lies not in the broad blueprints but in the strength of the coalition that can be formed to share a common vision.

The strength of a coalition is determined by the strength of the bonds that hold it together. Those bonds are as strong as the bonds between generations, between parents and children. They hold families together. Those same bonds supported the passage of Social Security to provide a degree of assistance in old age and the passage of Medicare, which freed families from having to choose between caring for their children and providing for the medical needs of their parents. We can build a system of care that brings flesh and blood to bear in the same way. Indeed, in many respects, we already are building it. In the process we will transform not just the care that is provided to the frail elderly but also the society in which it is provided.

Epilogue

Now sixty-one, I face with my twin brother and sister the problem of how to care for our parents. Most of our experiences are not much different from those of other adult children our age. Yet because it has influenced this book in so many subtle ways, it seems important to at least acknowledge the influence of our experience. Parents give us our first lenses for seeing the world. My parents' experiences as frail elderly persons have also given me lenses for seeing long-term care. Yet those experiences can't be understood, just as the facilities I have described in this book cannot be understood, outside of the context of their history.

Nancy and Henry were born during World War I, a few blocks' distance from each other in Catonsville, Maryland, but worlds apart. (My parents always insisted that we call them by their first names even as small children, a product of some utopian democratic vision fostered in the Depression that never quite caught on.)

Nancy was born into Baltimore society, the product of the union of the rebellious daughter of a successful entrepreneur (or robber baron in the language of the time) and the son of a nineteenth-century utopian socialist community. The entrepreneur's only mark on the twenty-first century is a toxic waste site, and the utopian community is now marked by only by a few piles of stone rubble in an upper-income housing development in Red Bank, New Jersey. Nancy's uncle on her father's side, Alexander Woollcott, terrorized New York City as a theater critic, radio personality, and participant in the vicious circle that met at the Algonquin Hotel in the 1920s. Other than the periodic revival of *The Man Who Came to Dinner*, a play parodying him, he also has left no mark.

Henry was born into a working-class family in Catonsville; his father was a day laborer, and his mother died when he was eight. Two maiden aunts raised him and his four brothers. A diligent student, he was able to attend St. John's College on a full scholarship and eventually receive a Ph.D. in psychology from Johns Hopkins.

My emotional connection to my parents was formed at childhood bedtimes. Henry was a storyteller who would tell stories about his own childhood and his experience as a young man sailing to Galveston on an oil tanker. Sometimes he would make up stories that were elaborations of the pulp fiction he read as a child about heroic individuals who survived and flourished in the wilderness with nothing but "a pair of BVDs and a pen knife." Nancy was a reader who loved the sound of language. She would read us poems and had a wonderful soothing way with the words even though as children we couldn't begin to understand them. This was especially useful when I couldn't fall asleep or was awakened by a nightmare.

Henry got a permanent faculty position at Michigan State College in 1949, and we settled in East Lansing. Nancy started writing and eventually published four children's books, mystery stories developed from some of our experiences as children. With other faculty who lacked housing in a rapidly expanding academic community, they formed a cooperative, purchased some farmland, hired an architect, and built, with the help of the sweat equity of the families involved, their own housing development. There was a closeness sparked by this cooperative effort. Neighbors, drawn from all parts of the United States and the world, felt nothing about dropping in unannounced on each other and organizing intergenerational pickup volleyball or touch football games and barbecues.

Henry built his dream retirement house on Martha's Vineyard in the 1970s, while land was still cheap and before it had become the visible destination of the rich and famous. Nancy's grandfather had originated the island connection with the purchase of a summerhouse on Martha's Vineyard in the 1920s. That house became known as "The House of Shattered Dreams." His dream was that his expanding extended family would join him there in the summers. The dream shattered when they did. Two of Nancy's three sisters ended up raising their families on the island, and it became a regular summer destination for us.

Henry's retirement house became an extension of Nancy's grandfather's dream, a place for extended gatherings of family and friends. There were volleyball games, animated play with the grandchildren, and magnificent feasts with Nancy's fresh bread and family recipes. A room was added to the house to provide space for these events. It also became an extension of my father's Depression-era youthful dream of self-sufficient subsistence farming. I had sent him a book I'd found on a bookstore remainder table by a University of Pennsylvania professor who had quit in the 1950s and had built such a farm in Maine. The author suggested that, even though you could be mostly self-sufficient, you still needed a small cash crop and that blueberries were ideal for that purpose. My father ordered the blueberry seedlings the next day. He organized them in rows from early- and late-maturing varieties so that when they fully matured in twenty years there would be an ample supply throughout the summer.

In building and expanding his retirement house, Henry never got over the blue-collar notion that there was something shameful and unmasculine about hiring others to do your carpentry, wiring, or plumbing, an insistence we are still dealing with. He created a three-story tower with steep stairs and a deck on top for watching sunsets and catching a glimpse of the ocean. The roof leaks and the plumbing is impossible to fix. The house lies down a long dirt road on an isolated part of the island that requires an automobile for access. It has now become their assisted living facility and a nightmare in design for its frail elderly inhabitants.

My father is now eighty-eight and has progressed into the later stages of Alzheimer's. His walks and bike trips that in previous years encompassed miles are now limited to circles around the house. He has long since stopped struggling to write a book about his lifelong idol Thomas Jefferson. My mother is eighty-five, has had a stroke, and requires a cane. She is confused at times from lack of sleep but always very clear and intransigent about staying where she is and caring for Henry. We have finally gotten, under threat of institutional placement, somebody living in with them to provide the assistance they need. It is a fragile equilibrium.

Are they living out the ideal of the assisted living movement? They are certainly aging in place, maintaining a degree of independence, and taking calculated risks that few facilities could accommodate. Is it the best possible quality of life for them? It is hard to be sure. They have the things they need physically, but their situation lacks the rich and spontaneous social interaction that was always such an important part of their lives. Yet I can't imagine anything more satisfying for them anywhere else. I suppose, as my father would have said, you have to rank rather than rate your choices. My mother would find the polished and artificial surroundings of most newly constructed private assisted living facilities repulsive. Just as for other adult children, it is hard for us to imagine that the staff of such a facility could really ever connect to their rich, complex, and, yes, quirky lives. Any facility would certainly serve as a poor substitute for the diverse assortment of friends and relatives, now almost all dead, who were such an important part of their lives. They still love the land around them, watching the sunsets, and seeing the stars in the dark vineyard night sky. Neighborhood children and relatives now come and pick the blueberries that cluster like blue grapes in a seemingly endless supply, and my father still helps with the picking.

It is a fragile balance and winter is coming. Nancy reads to Henry sometimes in the evening when he is agitated. She reads some of the same poems she read to us at bedtime and when we were awakened by a nightmare, like this one:

> We are not sure of sorrow,
> And joy was never sure;
> To-day will die to-morrow;
> Time stoops to no man's lure;
> And love, grown faint and fretful,
> With lips but half regretful
> Sighs, and with eyes forgetful
> Weeps that no loves endure.
> From too much love of living,
> From hope and fear set free,
> We thank with brief thanksgiving
> Whatever gods may be
> That no life lives for ever;
> That dead men rise up never;
> That even the weariest river
> Winds somewhere safe to sea.
> Then star nor sun shall waken,
> Nor any change of light:
> Nor sound of waters shaken,
> Nor any sound or sight:
> Nor wintry leaves nor vernal,
> Nor days nor things diurnal;
> Only the sleep eternal
> In an eternal night.
>
> —A. C. Swinburne

Bibliography

American College of Physicians (1984). "Long Term Care of the Elderly." *Annals of Internal Medicine* 100: 760–63.
Arno, P. S., and C. Levine (1999). "The Economic Value of Informal Care Giving." *Health Affairs* 18(2): 182–88.
"Assisted Living Concepts Settles Securities Fraud Claims for $30m" (2000). *Nursing Home Legal Insider* 2(4): 2.
Assisted Living Federation of America (1999). ALFA Model Resident Admission Agreement. Arlington, Va.: Assisted Living Federation of America.
Assisted Living Federation of America (2000). "Medicaid Consumer Account Program: A New Model for Reimbursement of Home and Community Based Services." Fairfax, Va.: Assisted Living Federation of America.
Assisted Living Federation of America (2002). ALFA Ethics/Mission Statement. Fairfax, Va.: Assisted Living Federation of America.
Assisted Living Quality Coalition (1998). "Assisted Living Quality Initiative: Building a Structure that Promotes Quality." Washington, D.C.: Assisted Living Quality Coalition.
Auerbach, J. A., and B. K. Krimgold, eds. (2001). *Income, Socioeconomic Status, and Health: Exploring the Relationships*. Washington, D.C.: National Policy Association.
Baig, E. C., and T. Reiss (1998). "When a Home near the Fifth Hole Isn't Enough." *Business Week*. July 20.
Barker, W. H. (1987). *Adding Life to Years: Organized Geriatrics Services in Great Britain and Implications for the United States*. Baltimore: Johns Hopkins University Press.
Berry, B. M., and J. C. Henrietta (1996). *The Florida AHEAD Respondents: Characteristics of Florida's Elderly Population Aged Seventy and Over*. Ann Arbor: University of Michigan Population Studies Center.
Better Business Bureau of New York City (2002). *A Visitor's Guide to New York*.
Billings, J., et al. (1993). "The Impact of Socioeconomic Status on Hospital Use in New York City." *Health Affairs* 12(1): 162–72.
Bodenheimer, T. (1999). "Long-Term Care for the Frail Elderly: The On Lok Model." *New England Journal of Medicine* 341(17): 1324–38.
Boyer, R. (1987). *Retirement Places Rated*. Chicago: Rand McNally & Co.

Bredin, K., et al. (1995). "Decline in Quality of Life for Patients with Severe Dementia Following a Ward Merger." *International Journal of Geriatric Psychiatry* 10(11): 967–73.

Brunner, E. (1996). "The Social and Biological Basis of Cardiovascular Disease in Office Workers." In *Health and Social Organization: Towards a Health Policy for the Twenty-First Century*, ed. D. Blane, E. Brunner, and R. Wilkinson. London: Routledge.

Burns, L. R., et al. (2000). "The Fall of the House of Aherf: The Allegheny Bankruptcy." *Health Affairs* 19(1): 7–41.

Burrows, E. G., and M. Wallace (1999). *Gotham: A History of New York City to 1898*. New York: Oxford University Press.

Burst, H. V. (1987). "Issues and Concerns of Healthy Pregnant Women." *Public Health Reports* 102 (July/August): 57–61.

Cantor, J., et al. (1998). *Health Care in New York City: Service Providers' Response to an Emerging Market*. Washington, D.C.: Urban Institute.

Chapin, R., and D. Dobbs-Kepper (2001). "Aging in Place in Assisted Living: Philosophy versus Policy." *Gerontologist* 41(1): 43–50.

Chipperfield, J. G., et al. (1999). "Primary and Secondary Control-Enhancing Strategies: Implications for Health in Later Life." *Journal of Aging and Health* 11(4): 517.

Claritas (1998). Demographic Projections for New York City.

Clifford J. L. (2002). "Voiceless, Defenseless, and a Source of Cash." *New York Times* (April 30): A1, B5.

Cohen, E. S. (1986). "Legislative and Educational Alternatives to Judicial Remedy for the Transfer Trauma Dilemma." *American Journal of Law and Medicine* 11: 405–32.

"Company Briefs" (2001). *New York Times* (Oct. 6): Sect. C, p. 3, col. 1.

"Compassion Pays" (1997). *Forbes* 59: 86.

Daniels, N., et al. (2000). "Justice Is Good for Our Health." *Boston Review* 25(1): 4–9.

Dobson, A. (2000). *Briefing Chartbook on the Effect of the Balanced Budget Act of 1997 and on the Balanced Budget Refinement Act of 1999 on Medicare Payments to Skilled Nursing Facilities*. Washington, D.C.: Lewin Group.

Eberhardt, M., et al. (2001). *Urban and Rural Health Chartbook: Health, United States, 2001*. Hyattsville, Md.: National Center for Health Statistics.

Federal Interagency Forum on Aging Related Statistics (2000). *Older Americans 2000: Key Indicators of Well-Being*. Hyattsville, Md.: Federal Interagency Forum on Aging Related Statistics.

Ferrasis, M. (1996). *History of Hermeneutics*. Atlantic Highlands, N.J.: Humanities Press.

Freidman, S. B., et al. (1995). "Increased Fall Rates in Nursing Home Residents after Relocation to a New Facility." *Journal of the American Geriatrics Society* 13(11): 1237–42.

Frey, W. H. (1995). "Elderly Demographic Profiles of the U.S. States: Impacts of 'New Elderly Births,' Migration, and Immigration." *Gerontologist* 35(6): 761–70.

Fulman, R. (1999). "Lazard Problems: Investors Look for a Way Out: Lazard's Ouster of Arthur Solomon Spurs the Action." *Pensions and Investments* (July 12): 2.

Bibliography 193

Gabrel, C. S. (2000). *An Overview of Nursing Home Facilities: Data from the 1997 Nursing Home Survey.* Hyattsville, Md.: National Center for Health Statistics.

Galbraith, J. K. (1998). *Created Unequal: The Crisis in American Pay.* New York: The Free Press.

Goodnough, A. (1994). "The Neediest Cases: An Array of Troubles Affect the Elderly Poor." *New York Times* (December 4): Sect. 1, p. 56.

Grob, G. N. (1994). "Mad, Homeless, and Unwanted: A History of the Care of the Chronic Mentally Ill in America." *Psychiatric Clinics of North America* 17(3): 541–58.

Haberman, C. (2000). "Joy and Anger as a Career Takes Flight." *New York Times* (April 17): B1.

Hall, M. J., and J. R. Popovic (2000). *1998 Summary: National Hospital Discharge Survey.* Hyattsville, Md.: National Center for Health Statistics.

Harper, B. (2001). Where to Have Your Baby: Birthing Centers. Lamaze.com.

Health Care Financing Administration (1997a). *Data from the Office of National Health Statistics: National Health Expenditures by Source of Funds, Calendar Year 1995.* Washington, D.C.: Department of Health and Human Services.

Health Care Financing Administration (1997b). *Summary of HCFA-2082 Tables, FY 1995.*

Hearthstone (2002). Hearthstone at the Esplanade. www.thehearth.org.

Hoffman, F. L. (1908). "The Problem of Poverty and Pensions in Old Age." *American Journal of Sociology* 14(2): 182–96.

Hogan, T. D., and D. N. Steimes (1992). "Take the Money and Sun: Elderly Migration as a Consequence of Gains in Unaffordable Housing Markets." *Social Sciences* 47(4): s197–s203.

Hokenstad, A., et al. (1998). *Medicaid Home Care Service in New York City.* New York: United Hospital Fund.

Holahan, J., et al. (1998). *Health Policy for the Low-Income Population: Major Findings from the Assessing the New Federalism Case Studies.* Washington, D.C.: Urban Institute.

"Home Care 'Saves' 29 City Hospitals" (1950). *New York Times* (January 6): Sect. 1, p. 33.

House, J. S., et al. (2000). "Excess Mortality among Urban Residents: How Much, for Whom, and Why?" *American Journal of Public Health* 90(12): 1898–904.

House, J. S., and D. R. Williams (2000). "Understanding and Reducing Socioeconomic and Racial/Ethnic Disparities in Health." In *Promoting Health: Intervention Strategies from Social and Behavioral Research*, ed. B. D. Sedley and S. L. Syme. Washington, D.C.: National Academy Press.

Hunt, M., and G. Gunter Hunt (1985). "Naturally Occurring Retirement Communities." *Journal of Housing for the Elderly* 3(3/4): 3–21.

Institute of Medicine (1999). *To Err Is Human: Building a Safer Health System.* Ed. L. T. Kohn, J. M. Corrigan, and M. S. Donaldson. Washington, D.C.: National Academy Press.

Institute of Medicine (2001). *Crossing the Quality Chasm: A New Health System for the*

Twenty-First Century. Washington, D.C.: National Academy Press for the Institute of Medicine.

"Is Time Running Out for Some Financially Troubled Providers?" (2001). *Senior Care Investor* 13: 1–4.

Jackson, H., and K. Acks (2000). *The Assisted Living Market: The New York Metropolitan Area as of September 2000*. New York: Integrated Real Estate Services, Inc.

Jargowsky, P. A. (1996). *Poverty and Place: Ghettos, Barrios, and the American City*. New York: Russell Sage Foundation.

Jarrett, M. C. (1933). *Chronic Illness in New York City*. 2 vols. New York: Columbia University Press.

Jaspen, B. (1998). "It Comes in a Box: More Firms Use Off-Balance-Sheet Financing Techniques." *Modern Health Care* (March 2): 76.

Jensen, D. (1987). "Whether Prison or Palace, There's No Name like Home." *Miami Herald* (December 3): Neighbors Section, p. 7.

Jones, A. F., and D. H. Weinberg (2000). *The Changing Shape of the Nation's Income Distribution, 1947–1998: Current Population Reports*. Washington, D.C.: United States Census Bureau.

Kallan, J. E. (1993). "A Multilevel Analysis of Elderly Migration." *Social Science Quarterly* 74(2): 403–19.

Kennedy, B., et al. (1996). "Income Distribution and Mortality: Cross-Sectional Ecological Study of the Robin Hood Index in the United States." *British Medical Journal* 312: 1004–7.

Kennickell, A. B., et al. (2000). "Recent Changes in U.S. Family Finances: Results of the 1998 Survey of Consumer Finances." *Federal Reserve Board Bulletin* 86 (January): 1–29.

Kihss, P. (1980). "Influx of Former Mental Patients Burdening City, Albany Is Told." *New York Times* (November 23): Sect. 1 part 2, p. 50.

Kihss, P. (1982). "Lag in Hospital Cited in Psychiatric Transfers." *New York Times* (April 19): B3.

Kim, S. Y., and G.-S. Hong (1998). "Volunteer Participation and Time Commitment by Older Americans." *Family and Consumer Sciences Research Journal* 27(2): 146–66.

Klaassen, P. (2000). Address at the Tenth Annual Spring Conference of ALFA, Orlando, Fla., April 14.

Knox, A. (1997). "Independence and a Pledge of Care." *Philadelphia Inquirer* (November 10): E1.

Koss-Feder, L. (1997). "Takeout Commercial Real Estate: Assisted Living Comes of Age: High Margin Market for Senior Housing Draws Attention of Local Developers." *Crain's New York Business* (October 20): 36.

Leavitt, J. W. (1983). "'Science' Enters the Birthing Room: Obstetrics in America since the Eighteenth Century." *Journal of American History* 70(2): 281–304.

Leiderman, D. B., and J.-A. Grisso (1985). "The Gomer Phenomenon." *Journal of Health and Social Behavior* 26(3): 222–32.

Levine, C. (2000). *A Survey of Caregivers in New York City: Findings and Implications for the Health Care System.* New York: United Hospital Fund.
Levy, C. J., and S. Kershaw (2001). "Inquiry Finds Mentally Ill Patients Endured 'Assembly Line' Surgery." *New York Times* (March 8): 1, 37.
Lindsay, J. (1964). "A 'White Paper' on New York City's Crisis in Health Care Facilities: A Program of Positive Action and Progress." Philadelphia, Temple University Library HealthPAC Archives.
Lobbia, J. A. (1997). "Thugs Say Landlord Paid Them: A Slumlord Saga, Continued." *New York Times* (April 29): Features Section, p. 2.
Longino, C. F. (1995). *Retirement Migration in America.* Houston: Vacation Publications.
Lowell, M. C. R., et al. (1900). "Public Outdoor Relief." *American Journal of Sociology* 6(1): 90–104.
Lynch, J. W., et al. (1998). "Income Inequality and Mortality in Metropolitan Areas of the United States." *American Journal of Public Health* 88: 1074–80.
Madness Network News (1976). *Madness Network News* 4 (October): 1.
Mahajan, G. (1992). *Explanation and Understanding in the Human Sciences.* New York: Oxford University Press.
Manard, B. B., et al. (1977). *Better Homes for the Old.* Lexington: Lexington Books.
Mancinko, J., and B. Starfield (2001). "The Utility of Social Capital in Research on Health Determinants." *Milbank Quarterly* 79(3): 387–429.
Manderscheid, R. W., et al. (2002). *Highlights of Organized Mental Health Services and Major National and State Trends.* Washington, D.C.: National Mental Health Services Information Center, Center for Mental Health Services.
Manton, K. G., et al. (1997). "Chronic Disability Trends in Elderly United States Populations, 1982–1994." *Proceedings of the National Academy of Sciences, USA* 94 (March): 2593–98.
Manton, K. G., and X. Gu (2001). "Changes in the Prevalence of Chronic Disability in the United States Black and Nonblack Population above Age 65 from 1982 to 1999." *Proceedings of the National Academy of Sciences, USA* 98 (May): 6354–59.
Masumura, W. T. (1996). "Moving up and down the Income Ladder." *Current Population Reports,* Washington, D.C.: United States Census Bureau, P70–56.
McEwen, C. A. (1990). "Continuities in the Study of Total and Nontotal Institutions." *American Review of Sociology* 6: 143–85.
McGurk, J. (2000). *Recruitment and Retention Strategies for Assisted Living Facilities.* Arlington, Va.: Assisted Living Federation of America.
McMahon, T. L., et al. (1997). *Hollow in the Middle: The Rise and Fall of New York City's Middle Class.* New York: New York City Council.
Mechanic, D., and D. A. Rochefort (1990). "Deinstitutionalization: An Appraisal of Reform." *Annual Review of Sociology* 16: 301–27.
Mendelson, M. A. (1974). *Tender Loving Greed: How the Incredibly Lucrative Nursing Home "Industry" Is Exploiting America's Old People and Defrauding Us All.* New York: Alfred A. Knopf.

Mirowsky, J., and C. E. Ross (1998). "Education, Personal Control, Lifestyle, and Health: A Human Capital Hypothesis." *Research on Aging* 20(40): 415–50.

"A Modest Boost in Housing for the Poor" (1998). *U.S. News and World Report* 125(5): 5.

Moore, J. (1998). *Assisted Living 2000.* Fort Worth: Westridge Press.

Moore, J. (2001). "Independent Senior Housing: Staffing Up and Making It Work." ALFA Spring 2001 National Conference.

De Lew, N. (2000). "Medicare: 35 Years of Service." *Health Care Financing Review* 22(1): 75–103.

National Center for Health Statistics (1975). *Selected Operating and Financial Characteristics of Nursing Homes in the United States: 1973–74 National Nursing Home Survey.* Washington, D.C.: National Center for Health Statistics.

National Center for Health Statistics (2001). Health, United States 2001. Washington, D.C.: U.S. Government Printing Office.

New York City Government (2001). *About the Department: Adult Services Fact Sheets, Single Adults for FY 1999, New York City Department of Homeless Services.* New York: New York City Housing Authority. www.nyc.gov/html/nycha/

New York State Department of Health (2000). *Medicaid Profile, FY 97–98.* Albany: New York State Department of Health.

New York State Department of Health (2001a). Nursing Home Profit Report Issued. Albany: New York State Department of Health.

New York State Department of Health (2001b). *SPARCS 1998 Annual Report.* Albany: New York State Department of Health.

Nursing Home Community Coalition of New York State (2000). *A Survey of Assisted Living in New York State: A Summary of Findings.* New York: Nursing Home Community Coalition of New York State.

Opdyck, S. (1999). *No One Was Turned Away: The Role of Public Hospitals in New York City since 1900.* New York: Oxford University Press.

Orr, J. A., and R. W. Peach (1999). "Housing Outcomes: An Assessment of Long-Term Trends." *Economic Policy Review—Federal Reserve Bank of New York* 5(3): 51–61.

Paradis, L. F., and S. B. Cummings (1986). "The Evolution of Hospice in America toward Organizational Homogeneity." *Journal of Health and Social Behavior* 27(4): 370–86.

Plsek, P. (2001). "Redesigning Health Care with Insights from the Science of Complex Adaptive Systems. In *Crossing the Quality Chasm: A New Health System for the Twenty-First Century.* Washington, D.C.: National Academy Press for the Institute of Medicine.

PR Newswire (1987). "New Housing Standards Set to Help Senior Citizens." PR Newswire.

PR Newswire (1997). "Lazard Freres Affiliate to Acquire Majority Stake in Kapson Senior Quarters for $250 Million." PR Newswire.

Preston, S. H., and I. T. Elo (1996). "Survival after Age Eighty." *New England Journal of Medicine* 334(8): 537.

"Private Hospital Loses Labor Fight" (1940). *New York Times* (July 2): 15.
Raab, S. (1990). "Neglect Found in Residences for Disabled." *New York Times* (August 6): Sect. B, p. 1.
"Regulatory Trends in Assisted Living: A Report from the Front Lines" (2001). Attendee discussion at the ALFA Spring Conference, Las Vegas (April 6). Recorded by Audios Excellence Professional Recording Services.
Roberston, C., et al. (1995). "Relocation Mortality in Dementia: The Effects of a New Hospital." *International Journal of Geriatric Psychiatry* 6(6): 520–25.
Rubin, R. M., et al. (2000). "Income Distribution of Older Americans." *Monthly Labor Review* (November): 19–30.
Salinas, P. D., and G. C. S. Mildner (1992). *Scarcity by Design: The Legacy of New York City's Housing Policies*. Cambridge: Harvard University Press.
Sapolosky, R. M. (1993). "Endocrinology Alfresco: Psychoendrocrine Studies of Wild Baboons." *Recent Progress in Hormone Research* 48: 437–68.
Sapphir, A. (1999). "'Black Box' Contributes to Nose Dive: Common Accounting Practice Creates Air Pocket for High Flying Assisted-Living Companies." *Modern Health Care* (October 25): 56.
Schneider, D. M. (1938). *The History of Pubic Welfare in New York State: 1609–1866*. Chicago: University of Chicago Press.
Schneider, D. M., and A. Deutsch (1941). *The History of Public Welfare in New York State: 1867–1940*. Chicago: University of Chicago Press.
Schökel, L. A. (1998). *A Manual of Hermeneutics*. Sheffield, U.K.: Sheffield Academic Press.
Siegal, N. (1999). "Owners Make Way for Tourists, Long-Term Tenants Say They're Left in the Lurch." *New York Times* (November 22): Sect. 14, p. 1.
Smith, D. B. (1981). *Long-Term Care in Transition: The Regulation of Nursing Homes*. Washington, D.C.: AUPHA Press.
Smith, D. B. (1999). *Health Care Divided: Race and Healing a Nation*. Ann Arbor: University of Michigan Press.
"The State of the Nation's Low-Income Housing" (1999). *Journal of Housing and Community Development* 55(6): 19–22.
Sunrise Assisted Living (2000). Form 10-K Annual Report for Fiscal Year Ending December 31, 1999. New York: Securities and Exchange Commission.
Sutton, J. R. (1991). "The Political Economy of Madness: The Expansion of the Asylum in Progressive America." *American Sociological Review* 56(5): 665–78.
Temporary State Commission on Living Costs and the Economy (1975). *Report on Nursing Home and Health-Related Facilities in New York State*. New York: Temporary State Commission on Living Costs and the Economy.
Thomas, W. C. (1969). *Nursing Homes and Public Policy: Drift and Decision in New York State*. Ithaca: Cornell University Press.
Thorson, J. A. (1988). "Relocation of the Elderly: Some Implications from the Research." *Gerontology Review* 1(1): 28–36.
U.S. Census Bureau (1998). *Selected Characteristics of Persons 15 Years and over, by Total Income in 1997*. Washington, D.C.: U.S. Census Bureau.

United Hospital Fund (2001). *United Hospital Fund Reports Severe Financial Problems at NYC Non-Specialty Voluntary Hospitals.* New York: United Hospital Fund.

United Way of America (2000). *The State of Caring Index.* Fairfax, Va.: United Way of America.

Vahtera, J., et al. (2000). "Effect of Change in the Psychosocial Work Environment on Sickness Absence: A Seven-Year Follow-Up of Initially Healthy Employees." *Journal of Epidemiology and Community Health* 54: 484–93.

Vallone, P. F. (1999). State of the City Address 1999 by the Speaker of New York City Council. www.council.nyc.ny.us.

Vise, D. D., and E. Bolstad (2000). "Seminoles Plan Gaming Resort for Hollywood." *Miami Herald* (July 6): 1A.

Waldrop, M. M. (1992). *Complexity: The Emerging Science at the Edge of Order and Chaos.* New York: Simon and Schuster.

Wallace, D., and R. Wallace (1998). *A Plague on Your Houses: How New York Was Burned Down and National Public Health Crumbled.* New York: Verso.

Warnes, A. M. (1992). "Age-Related Variation and Temporal Change in Elderly Migration." In *Elderly Migration and Population Redistribution,* ed. A. Rogers. London: Belhaven Press.

Waskerwitz, S., et al. (1985). "A Comparative Analysis of Newborn Outcomes in a Hospital-Based Birthing Center." *Clinical Pediatrics* 24 (May): 273–77.

Waters, M. C., et al. (1999). "The Second Generation in New York City: A Demographic Overview." Population Association of America Annual Meeting, New York City.

Wilkinson, R. G. (1996). *Unhealthy Societies: The Affliction of Inequality.* London: Routledge.

Index

adult homes
  conditions in, 19
  as contract system, 37
  defined, 18
  Farm Home, 155
  Harbor View, 99
  and home health services, 171
  in NYC, 86
adverse risk selection, 6
aging in place. *See also* individual case studies; NORCs
  in Assisted Living Program Housing, 143–45
  backlash against, 161
  and design of facilities, 173
  in Florida, 9
  as goal of assisted living, 166
  and insurance liability, 177–78
  as marketing tool, 177
  in NYC, 3–4, 85–86
  as philosophy of assisted living, 161
ALFA
  formation of, 60
  and housing vouchers, 175–76
  mission statement, 90–91
  model admission agreement, 181–82
Allegheny Health System, 75
Almshouse and Bridwell, 36
almshouses
  and Bellevue Hospital, 35
  and the elderly, 40–42
  and the Great Depression, 43
  as indoor relief, 30
  in the 21st Century, 78–79

ALPs. *See also* individual case studies
  as adaptive systems, 166–67, 171
  and aging in place, 72, 177–78
  bill of rights, 92–93
  caregivers as key to quality, 162
  as consumer movement, 174–75, 176–78
  defined, 18, 66–67
  and economic disparity, 167–69, 172
  and home ownership, 174, 176
  and insurance payments, 74–75
  and medical model payments, 77–78
  and NORCs, 86, 183–85
  precursors to, 69–70
  regulation of, 180–82
  as social movement, 78–79, 165
ALPS, business of
  cream skimming, 76
  financing, 86–89
  and liability insurance, 93–94
  and licensure, 135
  location selection, 84–86
  management of operations, 89–90
  and PACE, 68
  public funding, 178–79
  REITS, 75–76, 87
Alzheimer's. *See* cognitively impaired
American College of Physicians' Health and Public Policy Subcommittee on Aging, 52–53
American College of Surgeons, 94
American Health Care Association, 59
American Poorfarm and Its Inmates, The, 40

American Retirement Corporation, 88
Apt, Joan, xiii
Area Agency on Aging, 9
Assisted Living and Community Service Policy, xii
Assisted Living Concepts, 88
Assisted Living Federation of America. *See* ALFA
Assisted Living Program Housing
   aging in place, 143–45
   business strategy/market niche, 140–41
   care, cost of, 141
   caregivers' comments on residents, 142–44, 145–46
   caregivers' comments on the cognitively impaired, 144–45
   care, standards of, 145–46
   daily operations, 142
   and PACE, 140–41
   residents' comments on caregivers, 143–44
assisted living programs. *See* ALPs
Assisted Living Quality Coalition, 96
assisted living residences
   ARV Assisted Living, Inc., 63
   Atria Communities, Inc., 63–64, 65
   Atria West Side, 20, 182–83
   emergence of, 58
   Esplanade, 183
   in Holland, 59
   as investment vehicles, 61
   Kapson Senior Quarters, 62, 63–65
   licensing in NYC, 19–20
   Madison York Assisted Living Program, xii
   non-profit vs. for-profit, 160–61
   precursors of, 45
   Prometheus Assisted Living, LLC, 63
   Sunrise Assisted Living, xii, 59–60
assisted living residences, low-income
   Assisted Living Concepts, 88
   Assisted Living Program Housing, 140

City Towers Home, 146
deSales, 88–89
Farm Home, 155
Aster, John Jacob, 66
auction system, 37

baby boomers, 169
back box, 87–88
Balanced Budget Act of 1997, 57, 64
Bank Street College of Education, 12
bankruptcy
   Allegheny Health System, 75
   Assisted Living Concepts, 88
   CCRC, 68
   Enron, 76
   nursing homes, x, 64
   Vencor, 64
Barker, William, xii
Barnard College, 12
Bellevue hospital, 35
Bergman, Bernard, 54–55, 66
Beth Israel hospital, 14
birthing centers, 69
Blue Cross, 73, 94
boarding houses, 43–44, 83
Butler, Robert N., 10

California Teachers Retirement System, 65
care, adaptive nature of, 171–72
care, control of
   adult homes in NYC, 19
   and assisted living, 72–73
   homeownership, 173–74
   and the medical model, 50–51, 67–68
   and the medicalization of care, 71–72
care, for-profit
   and assisted living, 74–75
   City Towers Home, 146
   and early nursing homes, 44
   Harbor View, 107
   Health Campus Village, 119
   impact on assisted living movement, 131–33

physician-owned hospitals, 46
Residential Suites, 107
Suburban Manor, 111
Wall Street investment in, 61–62
caregivers
  CCRC, 68
  ethnic diversity of in NYC, 4
  informal, 174
  and the IOM report, 96
  as key to quality in assisted living, 162
  medical model of, 67
  and NORCs, 12–14
  PACE, 68
  as percentage of cost of assisted living, 90
  sickentroosters, 32–33
  staffing crisis, 179–80
  verzorgingsehuzen, 59
  and the Yates Report, 37
caregivers' comments on the cognitively impaired. *See* individual case studies
caregivers' comments on residents. *See* individual case studies
caregivers' comments on risk management. *See* individual case studies
care, history of
  almshouses, 38–39
  British Colony, 33–35
  Civil Rights Movement, 49
  Dutch Settlements, 31–33
  indoor vs. outdoor relief, 29–30, 42
  Jacksonian Era, 36–38
  and poverty in NYC, 28–29
  Revolutionary War era, 35–36
care, non-profit
  American Association for Homes for the Aged, 59
  early nursing homes in NYC, 46
  Green Acres Apartments, 150
  Shady Oaks, 126
case studies, private pay. *See* Harbor View; Health Campus Village; Residential Suites; Shady Oaks; Suburban Manor
case studies, public pay. *See* Assisted Living Program Housing; City Towers Home; Farm Home; Green Acres Apartments; Senior Apartments
CCRC, 68, 122
Center for Medicare Education, xii
chaos theory, x–xi
Chasson, Marlene, xii
Cherkasky, Martin, 48
Children's Act of 1875, 39
Children's Aid Society, 39
City Home, 45
City Towers Home
  aging in place, 148–49
  business strategy/market niche, 146–47
  care, cost of, 147
  caregivers' comments on the cognitively impaired, 150
  caregivers' comments on risk management, 148–49
  care, standards of, 150–51
  daily operations, 147–48
  residents' comments on facility, 148
Civil Rights Movement, 49
co-ops, 17–18, 86
Coalition of Institutionalized Aged and Disabled, xii
cognitively impaired. *See also* individual case studies
  and cost control of services, 30–31
  deinstitutionalization of, 53–54
  and GOMER, 21, 172
  homelessness in NYC, 20–21
  poverty in NYC, 17
  reform movement, 39–40
  and segregation among the elderly, 161–62
  transfer trauma, 71
Coler Memorial hospital, 21
Columbia University, 12

Columbia University School of Public Health, xii
Commission on Accreditation of Rehabilitation Facilities, 94
Commission on Old Age Security, 42
Commission on Quality of Care for the Mentally Disabled, 54
Commissions of Public Charities, 39
Commonwealth Fund, xi
condominiums, 7, 17–18
continuing care retirement communities (CCRC), 68, 122
contract system, 37
Cottage Colony, 45
cream skimming
    and assisted living, 76
    in Broward County, 9
    in Florida, 6–7
    and PACE, 68
Creedmore State Hospital, 184
Crimson Edge: Older Women Writing, 13

Darling v. Charleston Community Hospital, 95
deinstitutionalization, 53–54, 156, 184
dementia. *See* cognitively impaired
Department of Hospitals, 46
Department of Housing and Urban Development, 58, 140
Dix, Dorothea, 39
dog boarding, 24, 178
dually eligible elderly, 24–25
Dutch Reformed Church, 32
Dutch West India Trading Company, 31–32

economic disparity
    effects on assisted living, 167–69, 172
    and life expectancy, x, 27, 168–69
    as measure of care, x
    among New York State elder population, 26–27
1824 County Poorhouse Act, 41

Elizabethan Poor Law of 1601, 34
Empire State Home and Assisted Living Association of New York State, xii
enriched housing
    and assisted living, 161
    Assisted Living Program Housing, 140
    defined, 18
    Green Acres Apartments, 150
    Health Campus Village, 119
    Senior Apartments, 136
Enron, 76
ethnic diversity, 4
Evans, Harry C., 40

family care homes, 156
Fan Fox and Leslie R. Samuels Foundation, xi
Fan Fox and Leslie R. Samuels Foundation Assisted Living Project, xii
Farm Colony, 45
Farm Home
    aging in place, 159
    business strategy/market niche, 155–57
    care, cost of, 157–58
    caregivers' comments on community, 155
    caregivers' comments on risk management, 159
    caregivers' comments on the cognitively impaired, 160
    and the cognitively impaired, 159
    daily operations, 158
    demographics of residents, 156–57
Federal Home Loan Bank, 89
Federal Interagency Forum on Aging-Related Statistics 2000, 29
Fisher, Holly Michaels, xii
Fisk, Carol, 60
Florida
    cream skimming, 6–7
    rate of Medicaid payments, 7
    and real estate development, 7–9

statistics on elder population, 6
taxes and long-term care, 9
food stamps, 26, 139
Forum on Age-Related Statistics 2000, 24–25
Fox School of Business and Management, xi
Friends of Residents in Long-Term Care of Raleigh, xii

Get Out of My Emergency Room (GOMER), 21, 72
Getzen, Tom, xiii
Golden Rule, 95
Gordon, Mary, 13
Great Depression, 43
Green Acres Apartments
   aging in place, 152, 153
   business strategy/market niche, 150–51
   care, cost of, 151–52
   caregivers' comments on residents, 153
   caregivers' comments on risk management, 153
   caregivers' comments on staffing, 154
   care, standards of, 154
   daily operations, 152
   residents' comments on facility, 152–53
   residents' comments on food, 153
Guthrie, Arlo, 184
Guthrie, Woody, 184

Harbor View
   aging in place, 105
   business strategy/market niche, 99–101
   care, cost of, 101–2
   caregivers, 103
   caregivers as key to quality, 106–7
   caregivers' comments on residents, 107
   caregivers' comments on risk management, 105
   care, standards of, 106–7
   children's comments on facility, 104–5
   and the cognitively impaired, 105–6
   daily operations, 103–4
   demographics of residents, 100–101
   income disparity between caregivers and residents, 107
   residents comments on the cognitively impaired, 106
   residents' comments on facility, 104
Harlem Community Development Corporation, 89
Health and Hospitals Corporation, 22
Health Campus Village, 119
   aging in place, 122, 124
   business strategy/market niche, 119–21
   care, cost of, 121–22
   caregivers' comments on duties, 126
   caregivers' comments on residents, 123, 125
   care, standards of, 125–26
   and the cognitively impaired, 121
   daily operations, 122
   demographics of residents, 120–21
   residents' comments on care givers, 123
   residents' comments on facility, 123
   residents' comments on food, 123–24
hermeneutics, xi
home health care, 15–16, 30, 48
Horowitz, Herbert J., xii
hospice movement, 70
hospitals. *See also* individual hospitals
   accreditation of, 94–95
   Department of Hospitals, created, 44–45
   for-profit vs. non-profit in NYC, 22
   GOMER, 21
   and the hospice movement, 70
   impact of assisted living on, 132

hospitals *(continued)*
   influence on childbirth care, 69–70
   IOM report, 95
   occupancy after World War II, 46–47
   physician-owned, 46
   and poverty, 25
   as providers of assisted living, 119
   and Senior Apartments, 136
   statistics on in NYC, 22
House of Correction, Workhouse and Poor House, 34
Howard Hughes Research Institute, 65
Human Resources Administration, 53
Hunter, Kevin, xii

income disparity. *See* economic disparity
indoor relief, 29, 38, 41
Institute of Medicine (IOM)
   and NORCs, 184, 185
   and Shady Oaks, 130
   standards for care, 95–96
   and Suburban Manor, 117
insurance. *See also* cream skimming
   adverse risk selection, 6
   influence on long- and short-term care, 25, 73–75
   liability of assisted living facilities, 93–94
   and moral hazard, 24, 73
International Ladies' Garment Workers' Union, 13
International Longevity Center, 10
Internet, 170

Jewish Home and Hospital, 21
Jewish Theological Seminary, 12
Johnson, Lyndon, 49
Joint Commission on Accreditation of Health Care Organization (JCAHO), 94

Kaplan, Evon, 62
Kaplan, Glenn, 62
Kaplan, Louis I., 47–48

Kaplan, Wayne, 62
killer application, xiii, 58
Kings County Hospital, 54
Klaassen, Paul, 59–60
Klaassen, Terry, 59–60
Koren, Mary Jane, xi–xii

Lazard Freres and Company, LLC, 63
Lazard Freres Real Estate Investors (LFREI), 62–65
licensing
   of ALPs in NYC, 19–20
   of assisted living facilities, 180–82, 185
   of hospitals in NYC, 44–45
   under Medicare/Medicaid, 50–51
Lieberman, Geoff, xii
limited equity, 11
limited-licensed home health agency, 103, 171
Lindsay, John, 30
long-term care
   and acute care, 49–50
   effect of elder migration patterns, 4–6
   and emergence of the corporations, 54–56
   and public policy, 135
   transformation of, 169–71, 185–86
lottery, 32
low-income housing
   and ALPs, 135
   Assisted Living Program Housing, 140–46
   City Home, 45
   Farm Colony, 45
   and hospitals, 119
   New York City Housing Authority, 14
   and NORCs, 14–15
   and Section 8, 25, 175
   Senior Apartments, 136–40
   shortage in NYC, 16
   and SRO hotels, 17–18

Macleod, Bruce, xiii
Madison York Assisted Living Program, xii
Medic Home Enterprises, 54
Medicaid
  ALPs, 18, 135
  City Towers Home, 140
  deinstitutionalization of the cognitively impaired, 53–54
  Farm Home, 159–60
  Harbor View, 100
  home health services, 15–16, 30
  the hospice movement, 70
  hospital accreditation, 94
  housing vouchers, 175–76
  influence on long- and short-term care, 49–50
  the medicalization of care, 50–53
  PACE, 68
  payments in Florida, 7
  payments in New York State, 7, 178
  payments to nursing homes in NYC, 21
  payments to nursing homes nationally, 52
  payments to NYC residents, 23–24, 169–70
  resource utilization group (RUG), 56–57
  Shady Oaks, 127
  woodwork problem, 30
Medicare
  Assisted Living Program Housing, 142
  the Balanced Budget Act of 1997, 57
  costs in NYC, 6
  deinstitutionalization of the mentally ill, 53–54
  dually eligible elderly, 24–25
  the hospice movement, 70
  hospital accreditation, 94–95
  influence on long- and short-term care, 49–50
  life expectancy, 168–69
  the medicalization of care, 50–53
  PACE, 68
  poverty rates, 56
  reimbursements to NYC residents, 23–24
mentally ill. *See* cognitively impaired
midwifery, 69
migration patterns
  in British Colony, 33–34
  in Florida, 7–9
  between New York State and Florida, 6–9
  in NYC, 4–6, 9–10
mobile home parks, 8–9
Mollica, Robert, xii
Montefiore hospital, 48
moral hazard, 24, 73
Morningside Retirement and Health Services, 13
Mullroy, II, C. Patrick, 64
Municipal Hospital System, 30
mystery shoppers, 85

National Academy for State Health Policy, xii
National Association of Residential Care Facilities (NARCF), 59–60
National Cancer Institute, 70
National Civic Federation, 40–41
National Hospice Organization (NHO), 70
Naturally Occurring Retirement Communities. *See* NORCs
New York Association for Improving Conditions of the Poor, 38
New York Association of Homes and Services for Aging, xii
New York City. *See* NYC
New York City Department of Homeless Services, 20–21
New York City Housing Authority, 14–15, 16
New York City's Maternity Center Association, 69

New York Juvenile Asylum, 38
1950 Social Security Amendments, 47
1929 Public Welfare Act, 41
NORCs
   as adaptive systems, 96
   and assisted living, 86, 183–85
   defined, 11
   Morningside Gardens, 12–13
   New York City Housing Authority, 14–15
   Penn South Mutual Redevelopment Houses, 13–14
   and public housing in NYC, 11–12
Nursing Home Community Coalition of New York State, xii, 39
nursing homes. *See also* individual nursing homes
   as almshouse, 37
   bankruptcy of, x, 64
   as cost control of patients, 30
   current stigma of, 42
   Department of Hospitals, 46
   emergence of in NYC, 44–48
   financing of in the 90s, 75
   growth of, 51–52
   historic stigma of, 35
   and Medicaid reimbursement, 24, 49–50
   NYC statistics, 21
   as poorhouses, 134
   profitability, 178
   resource utilization group (RUG), 56–57
   scandals, xi, 55–56, 64–65
   statistics on elder population, ix–x
   transfer trauma, 71, 177
NYC. *See also* poverty
   as location for assisted living residences, 85–86
   migration patterns, 4–6, 9–10
   public housing, 11–12
   SSI payments to residents, 170
   statistics on elder population, ix, 4
   statistics on elder population, income, 23–24

Old Age Assistance payments, 43
Old Age Security Act, 42
outdoor relief
   and assisted living, 93
   and cost control, 30
   defined, 29
   and the Great Depression, 43

PACE, 68, 140–41
Phillips, Benay, xii
Pickard, Robert, xiii
poorhouse, 34, 93, 134
poverty
   after Medicare, 56
   and arson in NYC, 17
   control of in the British Colony, 33–35
   in the Dutch Settlements, 31–33
   governmental role in, 31
   history of in NYC, 28–29
   and homelessness in NYC, 20–21
   and hospital usage, 25
   indoor vs. outdoor relief, 29–30
   and life expectancy, 168–69
   and malnutrition in NYC, 16–17
   and the New England system, 37
   in the new Republic, 35–36
   Yates Report, 36–38
Programs of All-Inclusive Care for the Elderly. *See* PACE
public housing, 11–12

Reagan, Ronald, 60
real estate
   co-ops, 17–18
   development, 7–9, 66
   and LFREI, 62–65
   mystery shoppers, 85
   ownership and migration patterns, 5
   real estate investment trusts (REITS), 75–76, 87
   and rent control, 11–12
real estate investment trusts. *See* REITS
Reinhard, Sue, xii

religious institutions, 32, 44
rent control, 11–12, 20, 86
Residential Suites
   aging in place, 110–11
   business strategy/market niche,
     107–8
   care, cost of, 108–9
   caregivers' comments on risk
     management, 110
   care, standards of, 110–11
   and the cognitively impaired, 108
   daily operations, 109–10
   demographics of residents, 108
   residents' comments on the cognitively impaired, 109
   residents' comments on caregivers. *See* individual case studies
   residents' comments on the cognitively impaired. *See* individual case studies
   residents' comments on facility. *See* individual case studies
   residents' comments on food. *See* individual case studies
resource utilization group (RUG), 56–57
Richter, John, xii
Roosevelt, Franklin Delano, 43
Rudder, Cynthia, xii
Rush-Presbyterian Hospital, 69

Saint Vincent's hospital, 14
San Francisco On Lok, 68
Section 8, 25, 119, 175
Senior Apartments
   aging in place, 139
   business strategy/market niche, 136
   care, cost of, 136–37
   care, standards of, 139–40
   and cognitive impairment, 136
   daily operations, 137–38
   residents' comments on the cognitively impaired, 139
   residents' comments on food, 138, 139

tenants' rights, 137–38
Settlement Act of 1662, 33
1788 Poor Relief law, 36
Shady Oaks
   aging in place, 129–30
   business strategy/market niche, 126–27
   care, cost of, 127
   caregivers' comments on residents, 128
   caregivers' comments on risk management, 128–29, 130
   care, standards of, 130
   and the cognitively impaired, 128–29
   daily operations, 128
   and the IOM report, 130
   residents' comments on food, 129
Shattuck Hammond Partners, xii
sickentroosters, 32–33
single-room occupancy (SRO) hotels, 17, 21, 53
snowbirds, 5, 7, 8–9
Social Security Act of 1935, 43, 168
Society of Friends, 68
Solomon, Arthur P., 63, 65
Sparer, Michael, xii
SSI
   ALPs, 18–19
   Assisted Living Program Housing, 141
   City Towers Home, 147
   eligibility for, 25–26
   Farm Home, 157
   Green Acres Apartments, 151
   payments to NYC residents, 86, 170
   Senior Apartments, 136–37
   Shady Oaks, 127
State Care Act, 40
State Charities Aid Society, 39
State Commissioner of Lunacy, 40
Suburban Manor
   aging in place, 112–13, 116–17
   business strategy/market niche, 111–13

Suburban Manor *(continued)*
  care, cost of, 113
  caregivers' comments on residents, 118
  caregivers' comments on risk management, 116
  care, standards of, 117–18
  and the cognitively impaired, 111, 112
  daily operations, 113–14
  residents' comments on caregivers, 118
  residents' comments on the cognitively impaired, 115, 117
  residents' comments on facility, 114–15
  residents' comments on food, 115–16
Sunrise Assisted Living, 59, 61–62
Supplemental Security Income. *See* SSI

Temple University, xi, xiii
tenants' rights, 137–38, 182
Thomas, William, 48
Tobin, Eileen, 13
Towers Nursing Home, 54

transfer trauma, 71, 177
Transitional Hospitals Corporation, 64

Union Theological Seminary, 12
United Hospital Fund, 22
University of Rochester, xii

Vallone, Peter, 10–11
Vencor, 63–64
verzorgingsehuzen, 59
Visiting Nurse Service of New York, xii, 13–14

Wagner, Robert, 47
Welfare Island, 45
Willard State Asylum for the Chronic Insane, 39
Willard, Sylvester, 39
women's movement, 69
woodwork problem, 30
workhouse, under British law, 34

Yates, John, 36
Yates Report, 36–38

Zeidenstein, Sondra, 13
Zinn, Jackie, xiii

www.ingramcontent.com/pod-product-compliance
Lightning Source LLC
Chambersburg PA
CBHW030111010526
44116CB00005B/191